P9-DNZ-523

CONTENTS

FOREWORD

Because I'm an MD, I see countless diets cross my desk. Overweight patients come in hopefully, clutching a copy of the newest craze. My usual reaction? I tell them to see if the bookstore takes returns. I can't tell you how many crazy diets I've seen, from the ridiculous, like the cabbage soup diet, to the downright dangerous, like the high-fat Atkins diet, which puts the body into a precarious state called ketosis and severely limits fiber and vitamins. I even recall once seeing a diet that had followers drinking champagne morning, noon and night, while severely restricting food!

There are innumerable ways to lose weight. If all you want is to watch the needle go down on your scale, you can go on a starvation diet, take some diuretics, and be happy. Well, at least you'll be happy for the three days you manage to keep the weight off. Once you go off the diet you'll be adding pounds you never had before.

On the other hand, if you want to lose weight easily, never go hungry, have boundless energy and keep the fat off forever, there is only one sure plan, and author Tosca Reno knows it well.

Tosca is the absolute picture of health and vitality. She looks the way most women dream about, and appears at least ten years younger than her forty-something years.

But she wasn't always this way. No, by the time she graduated from college she had gained far more than the "freshman 15." Tosca found herself at over 200 pounds. While her weight went up and down over the years, she didn't lose the fat for good until she discovered "Clean Eating." Clean Eating is a lifestyle. You don't go "on" it and "off" it. You will find that your new eating lifestyle not only makes the fat drop off, it gives you radiant skin, lustrous hair and energy to spare.

Low-calorie diets will all allow you to lose weight, but what happens when the diet is over? You go back to the eating habits that made you fat in the first place. Then, because you've just lowered your metabolism, your body stores fat more easily and you gain more fat than you had before.

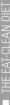

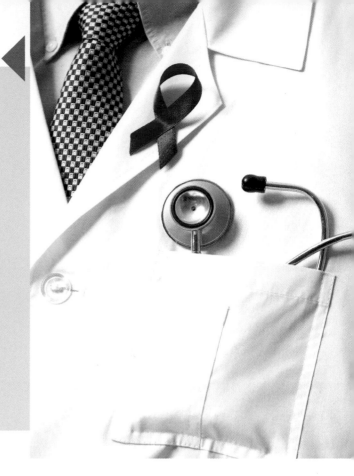

You will find that your new eating lifestyle not only makes the fat drop off, it gives you radiant skin, lustrous hair and energy to spare.

As well, like low-carb diets, low-calorie diets deplete your energy. If you have less energy, you use fewer calories. Again, this leads to future weight gain.

Eating Clean allows you so much food and so many calories that you will never feel hungry. You will have tons of energy. By following Tosca's eating plan, you will literally raise your basal metabolic rate, or your metabolism, allowing you to burn off more fat every day than you did before. Of course, this will help you keep the weight off forever.

The original and most famous Hollywood trainer to the stars, Vince Gironda, said that a great body is 85 percent nutrition. At the time many trainers scoffed at the idea, but it is now accepted wisdom (give or take a few percent) in the fitness business. As you all know, fitness models have to look fabulous all the time. Sure they work out, but if they didn't Eat Clean, all that work would be for naught. Now you can learn how they do it. Start Eating Clean. You'll never regret it.

Dr. Clifford Ameduri, M.D.

Dr. Ameduri is a well-known and respected physician who has devoted his life to the field of sports medicine and nutrition, with special emphasis on the physique.

MY INVITATION TO YOU

The Eat-Clean Diet was written for you, the confused but motivated reader who has struggled with weight gain and loss longer than you may want to admit. You may have only a few pounds to lose or you may have many, but you are looking for answers and a healthy relationship with food. More than that, you want a beautiful body! Everyone deserves that. In my experience the body is the greatest source of depression or motivation for many millions of you.

As I am a columnist for *Oxygen* magazine, readers write to me constantly with questions and stories about weight and body issues. Ninety percent of the time their questions have to do with how to eat. Since I answer every letter I thought it was time to write a book to help the many others who don't find the time to write. *The Eat-Clean Diet* book is my answer to millions of readers. I know I can help you because I helped myself.

The answer to healthy lifelong weight loss lies in the pages of this book. Eating Clean guarantees healthy, steady weight-loss success. It is not an elimination diet, so you don't feel deprived. Withholding food will not help you learn how to nourish yourself.

Eating Clean works because it incorporates healthy eating habits into every day. Almost as soon as you begin to adopt Clean Eating habits you sense improvement and a renewal of life. When I began to eat this way I couldn't believe the changes! Not only did I lose weight, I gained health and energy. I felt (and still feel) so good that people say, "Wow! You've done something different. You look 15 years younger." It is my sincerest wish that you experience this for yourself. Life for me is full of possibilities again, and here in this book you will discover the possibilities belonging to you. I will be there all the way.

A FAMILY STORY

In my childhood, meal times were an event – an opportunity for the family to come together. Although food was not the focal point, in a subtle way it was. Quietly, subtly, healthy foods were served at every meal, every day. We didn't know that the foods our parents served us were loaded with nutrients. We ate them because they tasted good. Not one of us was overweight, either.

Breakfast was always prepared by my father. The staple was oatmeal or Cream of Wheat, summer or winter. Boiled eggs and hearty whole-grain toast were the accompaniments. Only one teaspoon of sugar was allowed on our cereal. Soft drinks, packaged cereals and pre-made dinners were *never* part of the menu.

Today I realize how lucky I was to have been nourished this way. My mom was a genius at brewing up a pot of homemade soup, which was made all the better by the addition of my father's homegrown vegetables. Our meals were simple but completely nutritious. My mom, ahead of her time, often made lighter meals for supper. She understood that extra calories from a heavy supper would not burn off while you were lying in bed.

It was only when I lost sight of healthy nutrition and allowed circumstances to get in the way that I gained weight. This happened to me because I forgot to look after myself. Putting myself last was a poor choice, but as a young mother, I did what I thought I was supposed to do. I looked after my three young daughters and forgot about myself.

In some ways I feel I have been misled, too. When I went to the grocery store I believed that because the foods were on the shelf they must be good for my family and me. Obviously I could recognize that fruits and vegetables were healthy. These were always available in my house. Other foods enticingly packaged in colorful boxes were more of a problem. Nutrition labeling wasn't mandatory 15 years ago as it is now so it wasn't as easy to figure out if something was nutritionally sound.

Ultimately my life went off the rails. It wasn't until I embraced Clean Eating at the age of 40 that I got the body I thought only "Hard Bodies" could own. Literally from the very day I changed my eating habits I felt and looked better. It wasn't long before I had reshaped both my health and my physique. I could hardly believe it, but it was real and it was fantastic!

Now I am having the time of my life and I want you to come with me. At the end of my *Oxygen* column I invite readers to contact me. I want you to know I am always listening and so I invite you to do the same. Write me with your questions and concerns. I am always listening and I always write back.

In the meantime,

Eat Clean Today for a Healthier You Tomorrow!

Sincerely,

Tosca Reno

Tosca Reno

www.toscareno.com
www.eatcleandiet.com

Before, age 40.

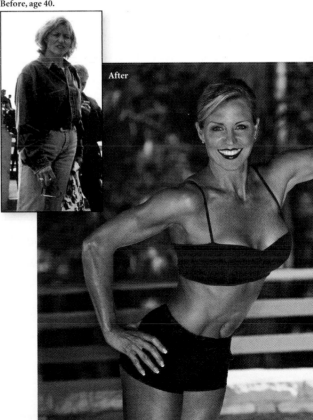

After

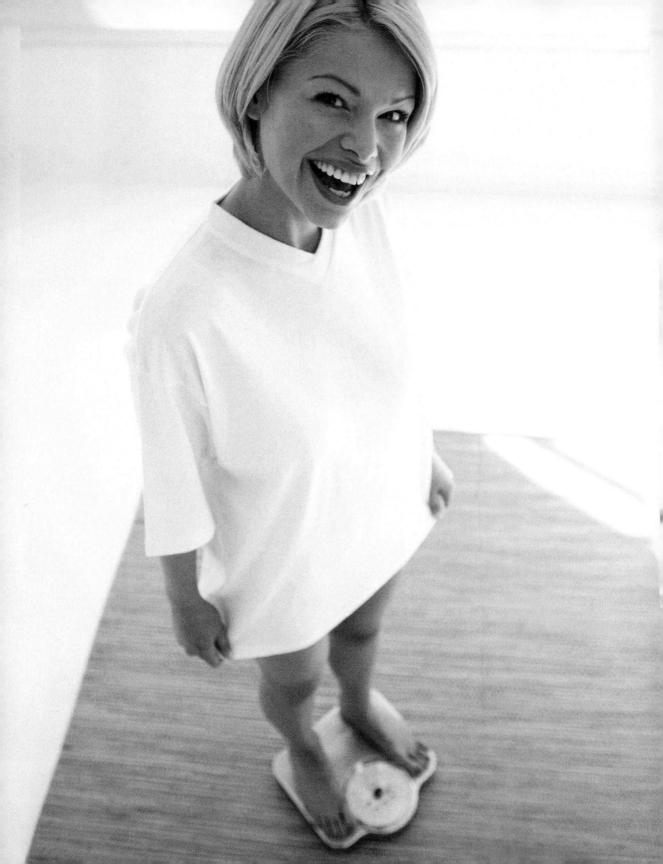

CHAPTER ONE

CLEAN EATING
A FUNNY THING HAPPENED

EATING CLEAN—
THE UN-DIET

What exactly do I know about Clean Eating? Clean Eating is not just a diet; it's a lifestyle. The commitment to this way of eating is full time. It's not about denying yourself or going hungry. It's about eating with thought and planning. Athletes rely on superior nutrition to keep their bodies tight and lean. Now you might not want to look like they do, since muscularity is an acquired taste, but everyone wants to have more definition and tone and less fat. By adopting the Clean Eating lifestyle your body will have a better chance at looking its all-time best.

DIET PROMISES

What kind of diet promises weight loss for life, plenty of food from all food groups and the body you have always dreamed of without costing you a cent? Can't figure it out? You're stumped because most diet plans want you to avoid eating one food group altogether. The Atkins diet wanted you to avoid carbohydrates but eat fats. Yes, you will lose weight, but that's just math; avoid one food group and you are taking away the calories associated with those foods so your weight will decrease. The truth is that none of these diets promise long-lasting results. Until now! Borrowing a page or two from the sport of physical culture, whose enthusiasts know plenty about trimming fat, the only way to do it is to EAT CLEAN!

By adopting the Clean Eating lifestyle your body will have a better chance at looking its all-time best.

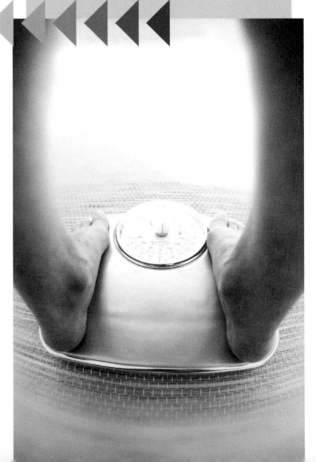

A funny thing happened to me in a grocery store recently. Pushing my cart through the produce section at a local supermarket I noticed a woman. There were lots of women but this one seemed to be always within my view. I had a distinct feeling she was following me as I was busy piling my cart with apples, broccoli, spinach, and berries, thinking of the delicious spinach salad I was going to make when I got home. The woman was watching everything I was doing. Whenever I put something in my cart she would wait until I had moved on and then put that same item in her own cart. Once I rounded the corner of an aisle piled high with melons and almost crashed into her. The surprise of the near crash finally gave her the courage to speak. She said, "Oh gosh I'm sorry, but I just wanted to know what you do to look like that. I couldn't stop looking at your body. You look so good."

Pretty soon her story came tumbling out. She was tired of being overweight and wanted to transform her body. She figured I must have a secret or two. "I have been watching you," she continued. "Don't get me wrong, I know it's funny for me to say this, but you have an amazing physique. Your back, your shoulders, your legs and arms are so toned. I want to look like you. How do I do it?"

Similar events have happened in airports and other public places. That's when I decided I had to share my secret. I motioned towards my cart and replied, "I Eat Clean." A puzzled look flashed across her face. She scanned my cart as if she were looking for Tide laundry soap. "What is Clean Eating? I don't

understand," she demanded to know. She was an overweight mother with two small children. It turned out that she had tried every fad diet there was but nothing had worked. In the grocery store that day I learned something important. I identified with that woman in more ways than she could have guessed, and I began to believe my story could help others. Not only could I inspire women and men to change their eating habits but I could help them make astounding changes in their lives and health.

HERE'S MY STORY

When the millennium arrived many of us were awaiting the predicted end of the world. Others were celebrating. I was cleaning my "personal house." To do so had become necessary, as things in my life had gotten out of control and rather messy. My marriage of seventeen years was failing, I was seriously unhappy and I weighed just over 200 pounds. No matter where I turned I couldn't get away from the glar-

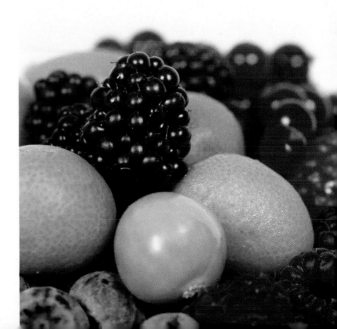

ing truth; I was a mess. The millennium seemed like a good time to make some serious changes. People from every corner of the planet were doing it and now it was my time to make a change.

First, a little weeding. I left my first husband, father of my three beautiful daughters. Trying to make the marriage work had taken its toll. We had been unhappy far too long. I then nurtured my brain with a return to school as a mature student to earn my teaching degree. My soul needed some cultivating. I purchased a gym membership and started to run. I drank copious amounts of water and ran so hard and so long that within a few months I noticed physical changes. When I stepped on the scale, the number blinking back at me showed I had lost 70 pounds, which were now in the dust somewhere behind the treadmill.

"No thanks! I've joined the gym. I'm taking care of myself for once and I feel good."

About this time I went to visit my doctor for my yearly check-up. I told her about the life-altering decision I had made to divorce my husband. She was already aware of the poor condition of my marriage. I will never forget the conversation we had that day. "Tosca," she said, "let me write you a prescription for antidepressants. You know, most women going through

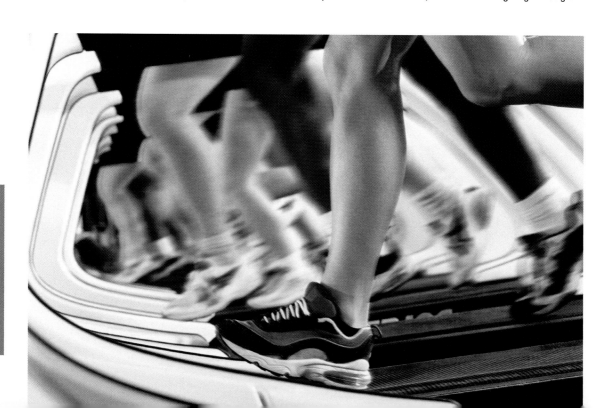

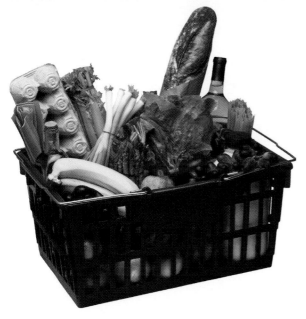

what you're going through need something to help them deal with the difficulties." My response: "No thanks! I've joined the gym. I'm taking care of myself for once and I feel good." I left the doctor's office without drugs. Seventy pounds slimmer I certainly looked better, but was only a skinnier version of my formerly fat self. It was then I learned the valuable lesson of Eating Clean.

EATING CLEAN — A LIFESTYLE

Eating Clean is a way of nourishing yourself that has absolutely nothing to do with soap, as the woman in the grocery store discovered that summer day. Try as she might to find anything else, all she could see in my cart was a colorful assortment of fresh vegetables and fruit, whole grains and lean protein. The backbone of Clean-Eating nutrition depends heavily on such food groups, eaten at regular intervals over the course of a day. Eating Clean requires you to give the big food companies, whose products live in the center aisles and end caps of grocery stores, a big thumbs down!

The most important feature of Eating Clean is what it isn't. Eating Clean is not a diet you follow for a few agonizing months, denying yourself certain foods. It's a lifestyle. Have you ever wondered why other fad diets like those you and I have already tried only worked while you were "on" them? It's simple mathematics really. If you usually eat PROTEINS and FATS and CARBOHYDRATES, as you should, and you remove one of those food groups from your eating plan, you'll lose weight. But only while you're on the plan. Once you reintroduce foods you haven't been eating during your dieting phase, BAM! You gain weight all over again and usually a great deal more than you lost in the first place. This is the phenomenon known as yo-yo dieting. In the long run the only folks who profit from yo-yo dieting are the companies who are selling the prepackaged foods you must buy to make the diet work.

INVEST IN YOURSELF

I want to make you a promise. Clean Eating is the only way to eat. It's an eating plan, not a restrictive diet. It won't cost any more than your regular food shopping (if you buy prepackaged goods, it will likely cost far less) and it guarantees results. I'll repeat that; it guarantees results. How do I know? Because I started Eating Clean many, many years ago. I lost the weight I needed to lose, created the body of my dreams and kept the weight off, all without going hungry. While I was eating my way to an improved physique, something else quite stunning happened. My health took a turn — not for the worse, but for the better. Much better! Before the millennium change I was overweight, but I also suffered from hypoglycemia, a condition where blood sugar levels are too low. One of my worst hypoglycemic moments was when I was in the grocery store (hey, we spend a good deal of our lives shopping for groceries!). I experienced a hypoglycemic attack while shopping and found myself passed out, planted facedown in the dairy case. Talk about egg on your face!

Clean Eating guarantees results!

had heaps of energy, enough to last me throughout the entire day. My interest in life, love, even sex was suddenly reawakened. Was it possible that I was a little bit sexy again?

I feel so good about life and the physical changes I have made that I want you to know the joy of it like I do. Clean Eating changed my life in such a stunning way. I am sure this is the way life is supposed to be lived. This book is written out of the passion I have to help you discover the only way to eat. I am like a phoenix rising from the ashes. Won't you come with me and truly live your life for the first time?

TOO TIRED TO CLIMB THE STAIRS

I also distinctly recall moments when climbing up a steep flight of stairs in my 200-year-old home left me breathless and sweaty by the time I reached the landing. What a pathetic state of affairs at such a young age – 35 years old!

Once I started Eating Clean many things changed for me. My weight remained steady. I no longer craved foods, especially sugary and starchy ones. My blood glucose stabilized, so that I no longer suffered from the horrible hypoglycemic attacks that left me sweating and breathless. My blood stats were off the charts – literally! I was so healthy there was no place to record them. My doctors were impressed. I

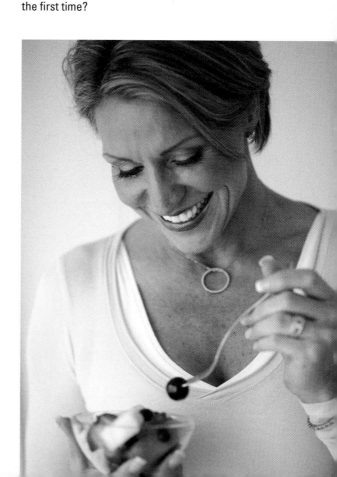

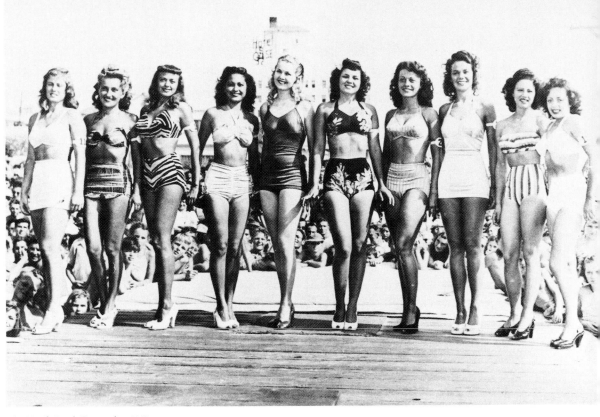

Miss Muscle Beach Contest, late 1940s.

EATING CLEAN—
A BODYBUILDING IDEA

Eating Clean is an idea about how to nourish the body which originated from a group of people who know all about creating a beautiful body. These people are physique athletes who practice bodybuilding, figure and fitness. Though these disciplines represent the extreme in the pursuit of an ideal physique, it is a perfect place from which to borrow nutritional practices, because they have to know what works the best. And every physique athlete Eats Clean.

WHY BODYBUILDING?

The cult and sport of modern bodybuilding became popular in the 1920s. In those days weight-trained bodies were jaw-droppingly beautiful, much slimmer and better proportioned than the overgrown, muscle-bound meat monsters we know today. Over time and with much experimentation, these athletes discovered how to reveal their hard-won muscularity by following particular eating practices. The last thing any of them would have wanted was a thick layer of fat that would hide the masterpiece they had created. What they discovered and subsequently followed was the Clean-Eating lifestyle. Every single one of them lived and ate this way.

EATING & MATHEMATICS

These lean, athletic bodies were shaped not only with weights but also with nutrition. And guess what? Great bodies come from nutrition far more than from weight training. In the fitness business, everyone relies on a formula that lays out the percentage of effort required in each category to build the best body.

It's clear the majority of effort in shaping a beautiful physique should be put into nutrition. One hundred years of empirical data gathered from hundreds of thousands of fitness professionals can't be wrong, and they aren't. Look at it this way. If 80 percent of your body comes from nutrition and you eat 365 days a year, then you might as well know how to do it right. Since physique athletes have tried and tested the practice for decades, it's safe to say it works well every single time.

HOW DO I KNOW?

Once I learned about Clean Eating, magical things started to happen to my body. A formerly fat and desperate housewife was transformed and finally had her lean moment in the sun. Pretty soon I was competing in physique shows, writing for a leading health-and-fitness publication and appearing on the covers of magazines. At 47 years of age! It sounds impossible, but it is entirely true. Who knows what

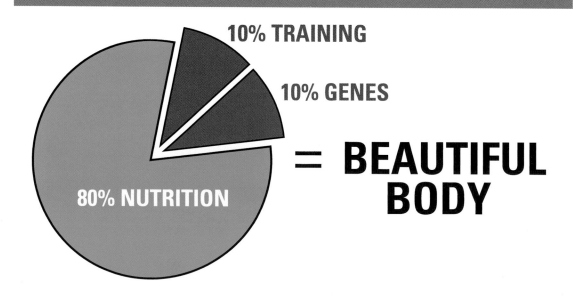

THE BEAUTIFUL BODY FORMULA

10% TRAINING

10% GENES

80% NUTRITION

= BEAUTIFUL BODY

GLUTEN-FREE CLEAN EATING

Life for those with a gluten allergy or intolerance can be very difficult. Gluten lurks in the most surprising places, such as soya sauce and bleu cheese. Would you think that phyto peptides are actually wheat gluten if you didn't know?

Luckily, Eating Clean is easy if you keep a gluten-free diet. Once you steer clear of foods that obviously contain gluten, such as wheat breads, the biggest problems are pre-packaged foods. Since Eating Clean already suggests that you stay away from these, you only have to control what goes in your own pantry. When you Eat Clean you need to eat food in its most natural state, including whole grains, vegetables and lean proteins. Well, vegetables and naturally raised meats are all fine for you, and the list of gluten-free grains is long:

⇒ **Amaranth**
⇒ **Arrowroot**
⇒ **Buckwheat**
⇒ **Cassava**
⇒ **Corn (maize)**
⇒ **Dried legumes and their flours**
⇒ **Flax**
⇒ **Millet**
⇒ **Nuts**
⇒ **Oats***
⇒ **Poi (taro)**

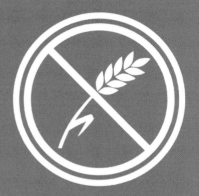

⇒ **Polenta**
⇒ **Potatoes**
⇒ **Rice**
⇒ **Sago**
⇒ **Sorghum**
⇒ **Soy**
⇒ **Tapioca**
⇒ **Teff**
⇒ **Quinoa**
⇒ **Wild rice**

I'm sure if you have a gluten intolerance you are already used to reading labels on everything you eat, so you are ahead of the game and should find it a breeze to start living the Clean-Eating life.

For decades oats were considered off limits for gluten-intolerant people. However, it has now been discovered that contamination by other crops is almost always the culprit, not the oats themselves. A few companies offer oats that are guaranteed uncontaminated with gluten, and the vast majority of gluten-intolerant people can eat these. While I don't normally use company names, I will make an exception in this case since this product is difficult to find. Here are four companies that sell uncontaminated oats: Gluten Free Oats, Gifts of Nature, Creamhill Estates and Bob's Red Mill.

lies in store for you? Whatever your Clean Eating future holds for you, you can be sure it's better than where you are now. If you adopt this lifestyle your body will have the chance for optimum health and for looking its all-time best, just as I have discovered.

CLEAN EATING PUTS THE ICING ON THE CAKE

Are you one of those people who exercises like crazy but never sees results? There are legions of folks like you in the same fat birthday suit. You scratch your head in dismay when you catch a glimpse of yourself in the mirror, confused as to why the exercise makes so little difference. Want to know what the problem is? It's your nutrition. No amount of exercise will reshape your body without appropriate nutrition.

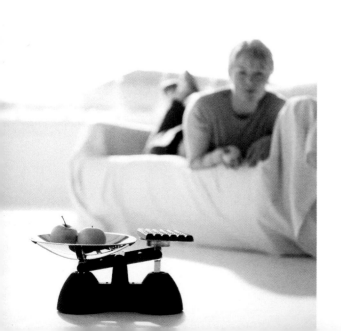

Picture a mountain peak, its jagged beauty and sharp lines softened by a blanket of thick snow. You can't see any of the rocky details underneath the snow. It's the same as the human body. Take a look at your stomach, your butt, arms or shoulders. A layer of fat obscures any muscle definition you may have, just like the snow on the mountain. Along comes a blistering hot sun whose energy melts the snow from the mountain. Sure enough, jagged detail comes into view.

The same is true of the clean energy you consume. The blistering fuel from superior foods such as complex carbohydrates, lean protein, fruit and vegetables melts away fat and soon your muscular definition comes sharply into view. That is the beauty of Clean Eating. Once you learn how to eat this way you will never guess again about how to build your best body. The rules are simple, the foods delicious and the resulting joy immeasurable!

80/10/10

Remember a beautiful body is built with 80 percent nutrition. You are about to learn what that involves, but you must pay attention to the remaining 20 percent of the formula. Your genes obviously play a role in your physical appearance. The shape of your nose, the width of your shoulders, the fullness of your lips and virtually every physical detail are yours thanks to your parents. Thanks Mom and Dad! To some extent you must live with these physical attributes.

Including weight training in my exercise plan made the difference in turning my body from ordinary into extraordinary.

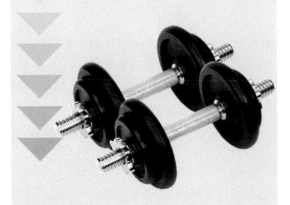

ENHANCE YOUR GENETICS

At the same time, you can make improvements to your genetic package by making improvements to your outward appearance. A thick waist can be trimmed down to a slimmer version; a saggy backside can benefit from uplifting resistance training and cardiovascular exercise; skinny legs can be enhanced by doing specific weight-training exercises to build them up. That's when the other 10 percent of our 80/10/10 equation comes in. No amount of Clean Eating puts shape into a body if it is not assisted by the benefits of weight training and cardiovascular exercise.

ADD THE WEIGHTS

Remember the seventy pounds I lost? When my excess baggage was gone I was just a skinny version of my former fat, floppy self. Although I had started to Eat Clean to keep the weight off, I had no shape. When I learned about training with weights a visible magic started happening. As a child my mother used to comment on how my butt was nothing more than an ironing board with a couple of bumps on it. My legs were painfully thin! I had a runner's body. Lean, but no shape. When I started adding fat to my skinny form I began to look very strange. Including weight training in my exercise plan made the difference that turned my body from ordinary into extraordinary.

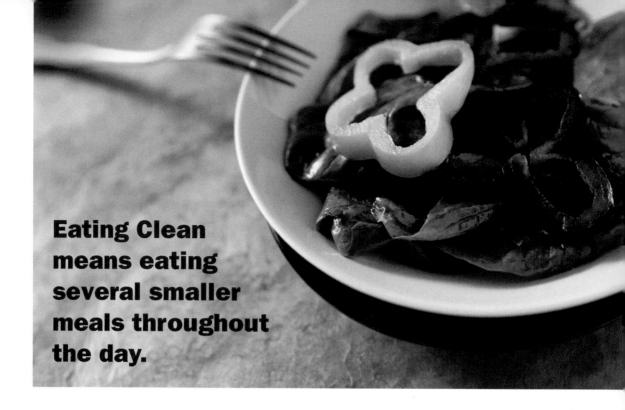

Eating Clean means eating several smaller meals throughout the day.

DISCOVER CLEAN EATING

The only way to continue to discover what this book promises on the cover is to act, and to turn every page with passion. Learn the rules of Eating Clean and adopt them into your day like the other good habits you practice – brushing your teeth and hair, showering and sleeping. Hey, if you made Starbucks your morning habit didn't that take some doing? You had to get yourself there, stand in line, order your drink, pay for it, pick it up at the other end once the barista had made it and then get on with your day. The same is true for McDonald's. The habits that got you fat and far away from your physique ideal also stole your valuable time.

CLEAN-EATING PRINCIPLES

So what is it all about? Clean Eating involves several principles of eating; principles which are as simple to follow as starting a car and heading to the gym or boiling water for tea. Everybody can do it! But are you ready to make the change?

You will have to eat more but make better food choices, eat regularly so you do not go hungry, throw out the junk in your trunk and brace yourself for the new improved you. Start by discarding the notion that you must eat only three meals a day and that the biggest meal should come at dinner. Eating Clean means eating several smaller meals throughout the day. By doing so you don't go hungry and your furnace, also known as your metabolism, burns steadily all day. If you do it right you won't experience those horrible "hit the wall" feelings that leave you reaching for a coffee or a chocolate bar. Dinner won't be the biggest meal of your day as it probably is now. Think about it. Does it make sense to fill yourself up with calories you won't burn off after dinner? Instead consume more of your food at the beginning of the day when you are more likely to be the busiest and have a better chance of burning the energy away.

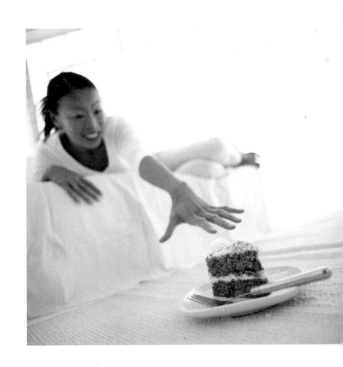

TOSCA'S CLEAN-EATING NUTRITION— *A TYPICAL DAY*

7:00 am	½ cup dry oatmeal (1 cup cooked) topped with 1 tablespoon each ground flaxseed, bee pollen and wheat germ, ¼ cup fresh mixed berries; 6 egg whites either boiled or scrambled; 1 cup green tea and 1 liter water
9:30 am	grilled chicken breast in whole-wheat wrap; raw carrots and cucumbers; 500 ml water
Noon	mixed green salad with cucumbers, tomatoes, carrots and peppers but no salad dressing; 1 cup water-packed tuna; 1 medium apple; 1 cup green tea and 500 ml water
2:30 pm	5 oz. lean cooked chicken breast, ½ cup raw veggies, 500 ml water
5:00 pm	½ baked sweet potato, 1 cup steamed vegetables, 5 oz. grilled salmon, tea and 500 ml water
Last meal of the day	½ cup low-fat yogurt with chopped apple, 500 ml water and or clear herbal tea

COMPLEX CARBOHYDRATES AND LEAN PROTEINS, A STEADY DATE

You may experience the feeling of lethargy that arrives around mid-morning or mid-afternoon, sometimes at both of those times. That horrible "hit the wall" feeling is due to falling blood sugar and unstable insulin levels. Before I learned about Eating Clean I always felt that way – sticky, sweaty, sometimes dizzy, too. I didn't understand why this was happening to me, but I definitely wanted to fix it. I didn't feel well. Sometimes it would hit me so hard I'd need to lie down and take a nap.

The answer to my problem and possibly yours if you can identify with some of my symptoms is to eat a combination of complex carbohydrates and lean proteins. Together they offset unstable blood and insulin levels by prolonging digestion and slowing the release of sugar into the bloodstream. The result? Insulin and blood-sugar levels remain steady and you feel better. According to **Lee Labrada**, super fitness guru and author of *The Lean Body Promise*, "By eating protein with your complex carbohydrates you'll slow the carb-to-fat conversion process even more." This is why you should never eat complex carbohydrates alone. Always pair carbs with protein.

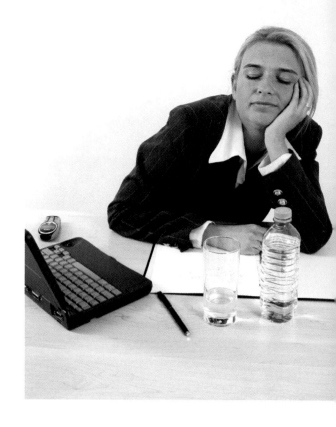

That horrible "hit the wall" feeling is due to falling blood sugar and unstable insulin levels.

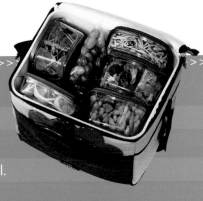

EAT-CLEAN PRINCIPLES

⤍ Eat 5 or 6 small meals every day.

⤍ Eat every 2 to 3 hours.

⤍ Combine lean protein and complex carbs at every meal.

⤍ Consume adequate healthy fats each day.

⤍ Drink at least 2 liters, or 8 cups, of water each day.

⤍ Never miss a meal, especially breakfast.

⤍ Carry a cooler loaded with Eat-Clean foods to get through the day.

⤍ Avoid all over-processed, refined foods, especially white flour and sugar.

⤍ Avoid chemicals, preservatives, and artificial sugar.

⤍ Avoid saturated and trans fats.

⤍ Avoid sugar-loaded colas and juices.

⤍ Consume adequate healthy fats (EFAs) each day.

⤍ Avoid alcohol – another form of sugar.

⤍ Avoid all calorie-dense foods that contain little or no nutritional value.

⤍ Depend on fresh fruits and vegetables for fiber, vitamins and enzymes.

⤍ Stick to proper portion sizes – give up the super-sizing!

>> >>>>>>

THE TRUTH ABOUT TASTE

Many foods dripping in taste and flavor, especially fast foods and prepackaged goodies, have been engineered to taste that way. According to **Greg Crister**, author of *Fat Land*, in order for food "to be convenient – to be stable and have a long shelf life, or to retain good 'mouthfeel' after an hour under the fast-food heat lamp – foods had to contain larger and more condensed amount of fats and sugars." That's precisely what food manufacturing companies have done; filled food with "stuff" to keep it fresh on shelves longer and to make it taste better. Unsuspecting consumers have taken the bait – well, it does taste good, doesn't it? Now far too many of us are overweight and suffering from disease.

This may get you worried that Clean Eating tastes bad, but nothing could be further from the truth.

Wholesome fresh foods burst with nutrition and true flavor. You will quickly develop a love for their wholesome goodness as you begin to cleanse your palate of your former food foibles. You'll begin to dislike the taste of the sugar- and fat-laden junk foods that you used to love. You'll feel energized and charged with mental clarity. Does it hurt that you're looking better?

PORTIONS – HOW MUCH IS THAT REALLY?

A simple way to get things under control is to re-learn proper serving sizes, something many of us have no idea about. No idea! How big should our lunchtime salad be? What's the right amount of cereal for breakfast? Should I eat an 8-ounce hunk of steak or 12 ounces? What does 8 ounces look like? When Eating Clean you must make a commitment to measure foods until you get the 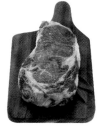 hang of how much you should be eating. You will soon learn that a 5- or 6-ounce portion is about the size of the palm of your hand. A serving of complex carbohydrates from starches or grains is the amount you can hold in a cupped hand and a serving of vegetables you can hold in two hands cupped together.

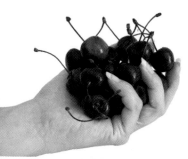

VEGETARIAN CLEAN EATING

I get countless e-mails about Eating Clean as a vegetarian. The good news is that there is no food allergy, sensitivity or food-avoidance issue that gets in the way of Clean Eating. However, some dietary concerns require a little more thought and effort, and being vegetarian or vegan is one of them. But if you're vegetarian or vegan, you're already used to eating with foresight, so this should not be a problem for you!

Vegetarians are often surprised to find they gain weight when they stop eating meat. They feel as if they are eating more healthfully and their weight should magically drop, and are shocked to notice their waistbands getting tighter! The usual culprits? Bread, cheese and pasta.

The key to success for a Clean-Eating vegetarian is the same key for everyone else: planning. For thousands of years humans have had to plan their food if they wanted to eat, thinking months and years in advance – growing crops, drying seeds, and preparing food for storage through long, hard winters. For some reason many of us now think it's okay to not think about food until it's time to eat. Well, my friend, whatever your eating issues are, that is a recipe for failure.

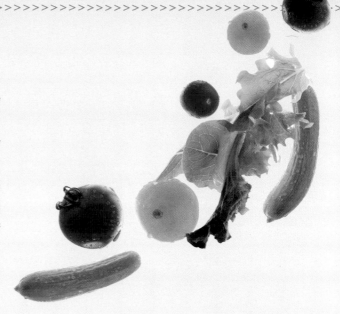

Vegetarians can have a hard time getting enough protein in every one of their five to six meals a day – which is where high-fat cheese usually comes in. The best way to succeed at this is to have plenty of protein choices on hand at all times. Keep tofu in your fridge and edamame in your freezer. Beans are best bought dry and cooked yourself, but this takes quite a while and if you haven't given yourself enough time or if your plans change, you could again end up without protein. Keep lots of cans on hand for such an emergency. Textured vegetable protein, or TVP, is perfect for recipes requiring ground meat. And a good protein powder is a godsend. Hemp and soy are two vegan choices. Quinoa is a superior food altogether. It's tasty, versatile, and it happens to be a complete protein.

And remember that protein from plant sources is usually incomplete. Even complete protein, such as soy, does not have the bioavailability offered from animal sources. If you think this doesn't matter so much, you should know that your body will break down your muscle in order to complete the proteins from your food! This is another reason vegetarians often find themselves gaining weight. Make sure to eat a wide variety of foods and to always eat lentils with whole grains and/or fat-free dairy, if you consume dairy products.

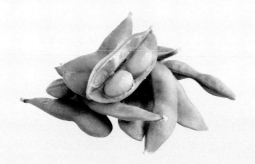

Nuts, seeds, and nut butters have substantial amounts of protein but they do also contain a great deal of fat. While this fat is healthy, you don't want to eat too much of it. Do include nuts and seeds in your diet, but watch how many servings you consume. One scant handful of nuts or two tablespoons of nut butter is plenty for one day.

Ironically, vegetarians often don't eat enough vegetables. While complex carbs from whole grains are necessary, too much will hinder your weight-loss goals. Keep to two to four servings a day of complex carbs from starchy sources such as potatoes, whole grains and bananas. The rest of your carbs should come mainly from vegetables, though a little fresh fruit is fine too.

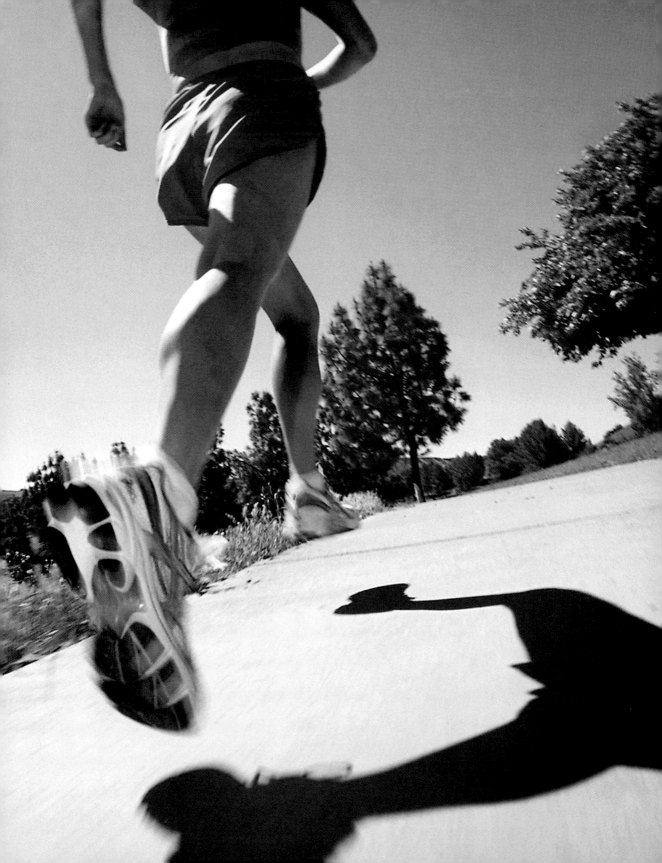

CHAPTER TWO

RENO-VATE
YOUR METABOLISM

HYPING THE METABOLISM

The conditions of overweight and obesity are often blamed on a sluggish metabolism. It's easier to blame a "condition" than yourself. The reality is that only a small percentage of the population can blame excess weight on a truly poor metabolism, although our own bad habits can certainly slow our metabolism down.

Metabolism is the combination of all physical and chemical processes taking place in the body. It is sometimes described as the rate at which the body burns fuel. Everywhere in the body trillions of cells work furiously to process the basic fuel components we feed them – *carbohydrates, proteins, dietary fat* – and break them down into usable fuel. That translates into energy we use to move muscles, breathe, keep warm and maybe even lift a few weights. The body is cleverly designed to withstand feast or famine, so

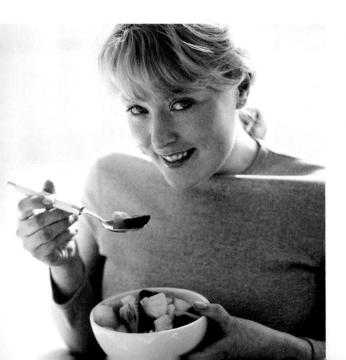

the metabolism is conditioned to burn hot or cold, depending on available food sources. Within a period as short as two days, metabolism can be reduced by as much as 15 to 35 percent below normal in response to reduced caloric intake. Sensing the onset of a crisis like starvation, the body slows down all metabolic processes as a protective mechanism.

UNIQUE TO EACH OF US

Unique to each of us, the basal metabolic rate, or BMR, is the rate at which the body uses energy when at rest. No one utilizes fats, proteins and carbohydrates in the same way as anyone else. **Dr. Philip L. Goglia**, author of *Turn Up the Heat*, states, "The body is a magnificent chemical factory governed by rules of cause and effect: what you put into it is what you get out of it metabolically."

An athlete who trains intensely and eats high-quality nutrition has an efficient metabolism. A couch potato whose only form of exercise involves opening a bag of chips has a sluggish metabolism. An individual who has dieted and gained weight repeatedly has a messed-up metabolism. The rest of us fall somewhere in between. We want to look better but find it hard to squeeze in a meal or a workout. That's why you're reading this book.

UNUSED FUEL IS FAT

Unused fuel is stored as, yes you guessed it, fat! The amount of fuel used to "run" the body varies from person to person as does the resting heart rate. The

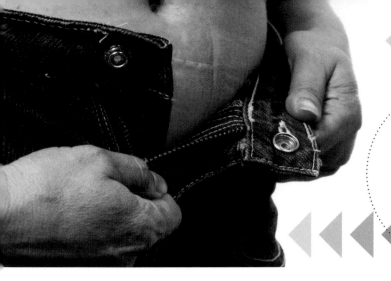

basal metabolic rate (BMR) is the amount of energy required by the resting body to stay alive. It is not a fixed number. The rate at which North Americans are becoming overweight suggests there is a lot of unused fuel being carried around.

INCONSISTENT EATING

One fact remains true. Inconsistent eating habits cause wild swings in blood sugar and consequently insulin levels. These problems are partly to blame for this new epidemic of overweight-related disease. Most of us consume only two meals per day; breakfast being the meal most often avoided. Other times, meals are eaten with so many hours in between that blood-sugar levels dance wildly out of control. When we eat inconsistently the body has no idea of what fuel to expect and when. Our BMR becomes sluggish as a result. Remember, it's trying to protect us.

A sedentary lifestyle is also to blame for reduced metabolic rate. An active lifestyle will increase it. This all suggests that it is possible to manipulate the BMR.

This is exciting news! If you knew you could accelerate your metabolic rate in order to chase away unwanted fat, wouldn't you do it? North Americans have forgotten the simple art of eating properly and exercising regularly. But it is completely within your capability to alter your BMR – either lessening or increasing it.

SIMPLE SCIENCE

Your BMR (basal metabolic rate) is not a fixed number. The rate at which it "burns" varies not just from person to person but also within the same person. Whether you have 15 or 50 pounds to shed, regular resistance training eclipses any other activity for jolting the BMR into high gear. The math speaks for itself. One pound of muscle burns approximately 25 times more calories than a pound of fat. Of all tissues in the body, muscle is the most abundant (if you are not overweight, of course). Since there is an abundance of muscle tissue and muscles demand more energy even when not in use, it is muscle tissue that determines metabolic rate. To speed it up you'll need more muscle. A more muscular woman burns more calories than a sedentary, unfit woman. The simplicity of it is brilliant.

TRAIN WITH WEIGHTS

Training with weights is one of the best ways to accomplish this, since a cascade of events take place in the body in response to increased physical activity. In a process called lipolysis, as soon as muscles begin to move, fat cells release fat and become smaller. Exercise also triggers the release of testosterone, another fat destroyer, for several hours after exercise has occurred. Resistance exercise also stimulates muscle growth and, if you remember, more muscle burns more fat. If the thought of training with weights scares you, don't let it. Unless women take steroids they cannot build huge muscles no matter how hard they may try. In fact, the women's bodies that you find most attractive and appealing were no doubt created with weights.

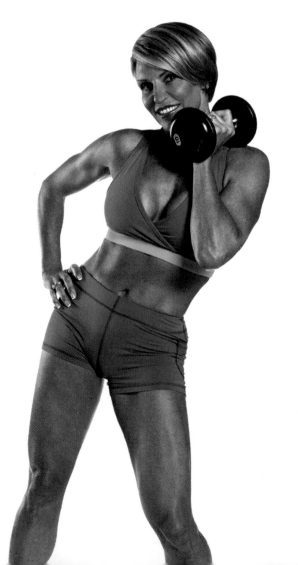

Muscle is effective because it chases away body fat and deposits muscle fiber in its place. Incorporating four or five lifting sessions into a week will produce the changes in your physique you've been looking for, not just an increased metabolic rate. Focus on training the large muscle groups like legs, butt, chest, and back. Training these areas acts as a catalyst for burning calories and increasing metabolism. With testosterone pouring into the system, your metabolism stays elevated for several hours after the training session has ended.

Strenuous exercise causes little explosions of muscle contractions, generating 100 times the normal resting amount of heat in a single muscle. Just imagine the increased overall heat production occurring in the entire body with hundreds of muscles contracting at once during a weight-training session! The metabolic rate increases as much as 2000 percent! With every calorie used as fuel, the body draws on its enormous fat-burning capacity. Building a layer of muscle tissue is a surefire way of increasing your metabolic rate.

INCREASE WORKOUT INTENSITY, INCREASE BMR

Another excellent metabolism-boosting strategy involves increasing your workout intensity. That means you need to put your mind into the muscle. Focus intensely on what you are doing when you grab the weights. Concentrate when you lift them and be there when you bring them down again. In other words, incorporate the power of your mind into each movement to maximize your efforts.

I often see people at the gym staring off in another direction while they work the machines. They don't appear to really "be there." That sort of attitude doesn't deliver great results. Some people may say they enjoyed the novel they were reading while they were on the treadmill, but their mind was on the book, not the workout.

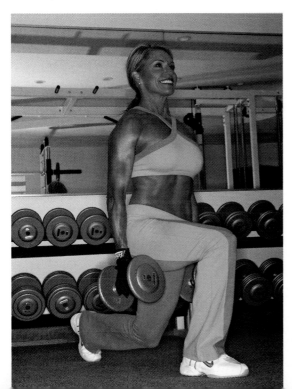

▶▶▶▶▶▶

Building a layer of muscle tissue is a surefire way of increasing your metabolic rate.

▶▶▶▶▶▶

INTERVAL TRAINING TO UP YOUR METABOLISM

You can also incorporate the benefits of interval training to maximize your metabolic boost. Interval training involves performing a cardiovascular exercise at the maximum level for a period of time, say, two to five minutes, and then dropping the level of intensity for the same period of time. Repeat the intervals for as long as you can manage. These short, explosive sessions serve to fire up a lazy metabolism. By adding two or three sessions of interval training to your mix of cardiovascular exercise and weight training, you fire up your metabolism – so much that nearly twice as much weight is lost among folks who do interval training than among those who don't.

Take it up a notch further by splitting workouts. Instead of training once a day, do a cardio session in the morning and a weight-training session in the afternoon or evening. This way you are stimulating your metabolic rate twice per day.

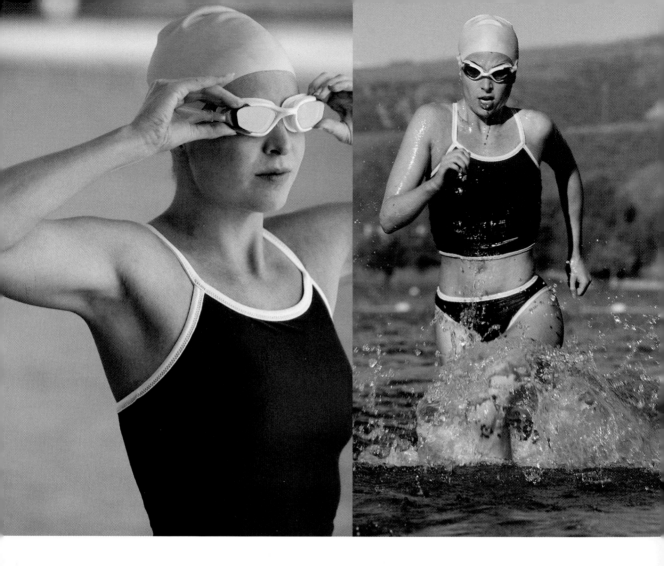

NO MORE YO-YO DIETING

One of the first things you'll need to do when considering losing weight is to give up fad, or yo-yo, dieting. Countless North Americans have been on one or more of these because we're diet crazy. Statistics show more than one-third of us are dieting every day. Yet 90 percent of these diets deliver no results. Sure you lose weight temporarily, but then you gain it all back and then some. Think about it. High-fat diet, low-fat diet, Scarsdale, grapefruit, cabbage soup. Avoid carbs! Eat protein! Eat fat. More fiber. Eat it all and get confused while gaining more weight.

Yo-yo and fad dieting only serve to tax the body by sending it into an unnecessary "starvation" mode. The metabolism goes into hibernation, preparing for scant food supplies. This is definitely not something we want. What's needed instead is food supercharged with energy.

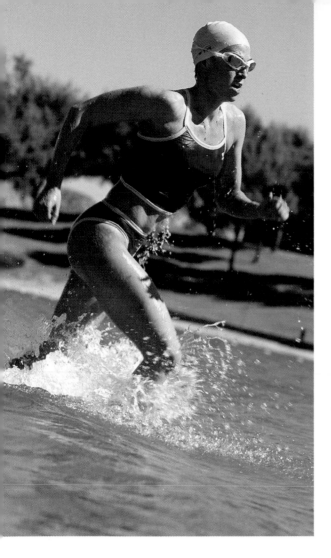

The body runs like a computer, smart and efficient. It prefers to burn energy from carbohydrates rather than fat, since carbs are more readily utilized. On the other hand, ingested fats must be first digested, then carried via the blood to every cell in the body. Fat doesn't dissolve in the blood like carbs do. When excess fat is consumed, your metabolic rate does not change. Instead the excess is, according to **Dr. Michael Colgan**, author of *The New Nutrition*, "layered onto all the wrong places."

WHAT ARE YOU EATING?

What are you feeding your muscles? To maintain a healthy physique you must nourish it with high-quality food, especially lean protein and complex carbohydrates. Otherwise, muscle tissue will be flat and your metabolic rate will be flatter.

SLEEP TIGHT

Our parents were right when they encouraged us to get to bed early. Only during the hours we are in a deep sleep is human growth hormone produced. What's that? Growth hormone works directly on cells to stimulate metabolism. It occurs naturally in each of us, increasing the metabolic rate by as much as 20 percent. It is much easier to stay slim in the younger years, since HGH – human growth hormone – is produced in enormous quantity, far greater than that produced even at the age of thirty. If you're constantly in a state of exhaustion due to lack of sleep you'll come up empty for energy.

These short, explosive sessions serve to fire up a lazy metabolism.

Human growth hormone is also produced during strenuous weight training. It is important to train with weights at least three or four times per week.

HAVE SEX!

The release of male and female sex hormones causes an increase in metabolic rate. Having sex increases BMR by as much as 15 percent. This is a good argument for enjoying sexual activity more regularly.

To maintain a healthy physique you must nourish it with high-quality food, especially lean protein and complex carbohydrates.

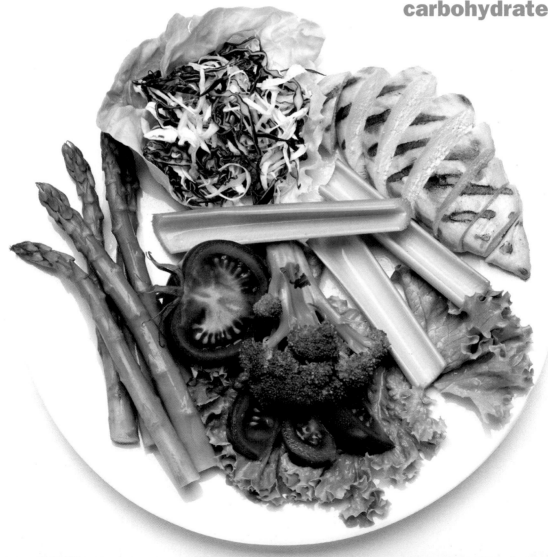

HERE'S HOW TO EAT
YOUR BODY ON FIRE

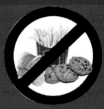

- **Toss simple carbs** out the door along with your soda-and-sweets habit. Foods comprised of simple sugars have a high glycemic index. This causes a spike in insulin levels, which negatively affects the metabolism. Too much insulin tells the body to store fat quickly and prevent your body from drawing on fat for energy needs. If you want to lose weight, you must make sure that your body's fat is the primary source of energy. In short, avoid the white stuff!

- **Keep meals small**. While this eating plan does not advocate calorie counting, a typical healthy diet consists of 1800-2200 calories per day; depending on your build and activity level. The Eat-Clean meals are small and consist of about 300-400 calories. Your energy intake is spread throughout the day and this will contribute to your weight loss.

- **Consume complete proteins**. This increases your BMR. The best sources include lean chicken breast, white fish, salmon, tuna, egg whites, turkey, pork and beef tenderloin, elk, and bison. The body uses up enormous stores of energy to properly digest and process protein. That's a lot of calorie burning taking place! When you consume protein with every meal instead of simple carbs, the body releases lipase, a hormone that makes the body rely on fat as its primary fuel source, instead of releasing insulin.

- **Complex carbohydrates** found in whole grains, fresh fruit and vegetables are a must for boosting metabolism. Complex carbohydrates are processed slowly, staying in the gut for far longer than a freezie. Blood-sugar levels won't swing wildly out of control, so insulin levels stay steady. Remember, too much circulating insulin causes the body to draw on sugar as a fuel source instead of fat. Plenty of complex carbs with a low glycemic index taste great. Just cruise through the produce section at your grocery store and reach for fresh fruit and vegetables.

- Some fat is required for the body to run properly, but it is the **essential fatty acids** – EFAs – you must reach for. EFAs accelerate fat burning. In the presence of essential fatty acids, cells burn greater amounts of oxygen. The more oxygen carried to the cells, the faster body fat is burned. Not every oil is an EFA, so be careful to choose oils like olive, flaxseed, pumpkin, fish oils and grapeseed oil.

- It is imperative that adequate **water** is consumed in order to help the body assimilate macronutrients*, vitamins and minerals and to flush out toxins. Without adequate water, bodily functions cannot take place.

- Supplement your diet with a **high-quality multivitamin**. It is difficult to get all the minerals and vitamins from diet alone, especially when you are physically active or under stress.

* **Macronutrients**: Food has two jobs: to provide energy and to provide nutrients. Macronutrients are nutrients required in larger quantities. They include protein, fat

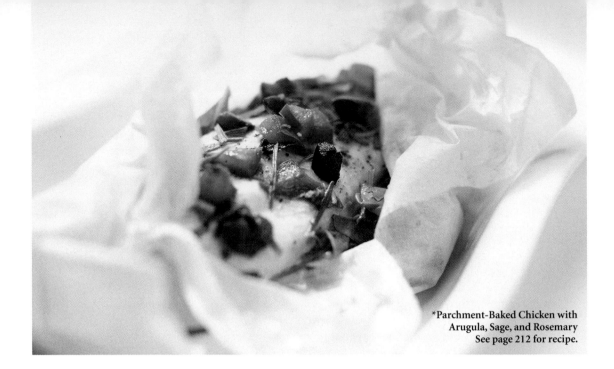

*Parchment-Baked Chicken with
Arugula, Sage, and Rosemary
See page 212 for recipe.

TURN UP THE HEAT!

Ever had that warm, fuzzy feeling after eating? That means your metabolism is running on high. When you eat a nutritious meal of lean protein and complex carbohydrates, a chain of metabolic events begins as food is transformed into nutrients. The warm fuzzy feeling you experience 30 minutes later is the result of heat released during the digestion process. Whenever heat is released, the metabolism is hyped.

PROTEIN INCREASES YOUR METABOLISM

Your metabolic rate increases when protein is consumed because the number of chemical reactions necessary to digest protein is higher than those needed to digest other macronutrients. This increase is brought about by the way in which amino acids, the building blocks of protein, stimulate cellular activity. Eating a meal loaded with carbohydrates increases your BMR only slightly. Eating a meal of chicken and carbohydrates causes your BMR to begin to rise within the hour, hit a peak 30 percent above normal, and last as long as three to twelve hours. Scientifically this is called the dynamic action of protein.

HOW BADLY DO YOU WANT IT?

Remember this, *"When man has had a hand in the manufacture of food, chances are it is junk!"* The sooner you begin to adopt the principles of **Eating Clean** the sooner you will recognize the truth of that statement. So now the only question you have to ask yourself is, *"How badly do I want to make changes?"*

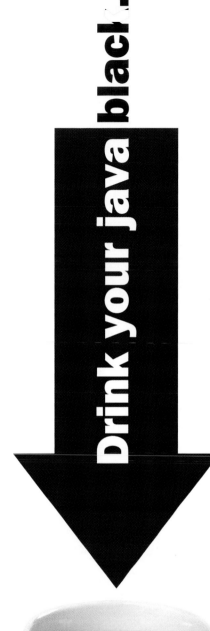

Drink your java black.

YOUR METABOLISM-
BOOSTING LIST

✔ Train major muscle groups at least three or four times per week.

✔ Quit yo-yo dieting. Lack of food snuffs out the pilot light that fires your metabolism, sending it into hibernation.

✔ Eat more high-quality foods.

✔ Exchange simple carbohydrates for complex carbs.

✔ Keep meals small, consuming 300 to 400 calories per meal.

✔ Eat at least six small meals a day.

✔ Eat protein and complex carbohydrates at every meal.

✔ Consume EFAs, especially flaxseed oil.

✔ Hydrate yourself with two to three liters of water per day.

✔ Supplement with a good-quality vitamin.

✔ Lift weights regularly, especially as you age.

✔ Eat spicy foods, cinnamon and turmeric.

✔ Drink your java black.

✔ Ditch the soda right now!

⑩ BEST METABOLISM-HYPING TIPS

1 **Water, water, water.** Hydrate yourself with water to encourage optimal bodily function and speed up the metabolism.

2 Eat a palm-sized serving of protein along with complex carbohydrates every two to three hours. **That means six meals a day, not three squares.**

3 Burn fat efficiently by **adding essential fatty acids** like flaxseed and unsaturated oils to the diet.

4 **Fiber fills you up**, sustaining you for longer than foods without it. Certain foods like flaxseed, wheat germ and bran stimulate lazy bowels.

5 **Vitamins and minerals** complement a clean diet, protecting against deficiencies and boosting the immune system.

6 **Don't go past the point of hunger**. Skipping a meal triggers a starvation response in the metabolism, making it slow down. Eating clean foods frequently sustains a highly charged metabolic rate.

7 Each meal should include a four- or five-ounce portion of **lean protein** from chicken, turkey, egg whites, pork tenderloin or white fish sources.

8 **Sugar is the white poison**, sending the metabolism into a slow tailspin. All simple sugars – refined sugars – must be avoided to keep the metabolism burning quickly.

9 **Complex carbohydrates** from fruits and vegetables satisfy the needs of an active body. Each meal should include generous servings.

10 Certain foods have a **high glycemic index**. This means they induce a similar negative effect on metabolism to eating sugar. Rice cakes, carrots, potatoes and fruit juices have a high glycemic index and should be **consumed in moderation**.

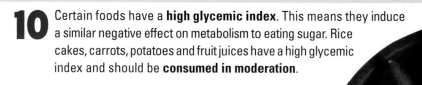

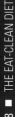

ENERGY BURNED PER HOUR OF ACTIVITY

Activity	Energy Burned (Calories per hour)
Sleeping	65
Awake, lying still	77
Sitting at rest	100
Standing, relaxed	105
Dressing and undressing	118
Light exercise	170
Walking slowly, 2.6 mph	200
Active exercise	290
Heavy exercise	450
Swimming	500
Jogging, 5.3 mph	570
Strenuous exercise, weightlifting	600
Speed walking, 5.3 mph	650
Running upstairs	1100

PROPER PORTION SIZES

1 serving lean protein = **palm of your hand**

1 serving of complex carbs from whole grains = **one cupped hand**

1 serving of complex carbs from fresh fruits or vegetables = **two cupped hands together**

METABOLISM & STRENGTH TRAINING

- Incorporate at least three, 30-minute strength-training workouts per week. Do 3 sets of 10-15 reps for each exercise.

- Don't select overly heavy weights, especially when you're just beginning. The general rule of thumb is if you can easily do the last few reps in a set, the weight is too light.

- Muscles are the only place where the body burns fuel, namely fat and carbohydrates.

- Metabolic rate drops about 10 calories a day per year starting at age 35. The amount of muscle in a woman (or man) also begins dropping at that age.

- Each pound of muscle burns approximately 50 calories a day.

- Each pound of fat burns approximately 2 calories a day.

- Fat takes up at least three times the volume of muscle.

- That explains why a woman with little muscle who weighs 120 pounds (a skinny number in most people's minds) looks worse than a muscular woman weighing 140 pounds.

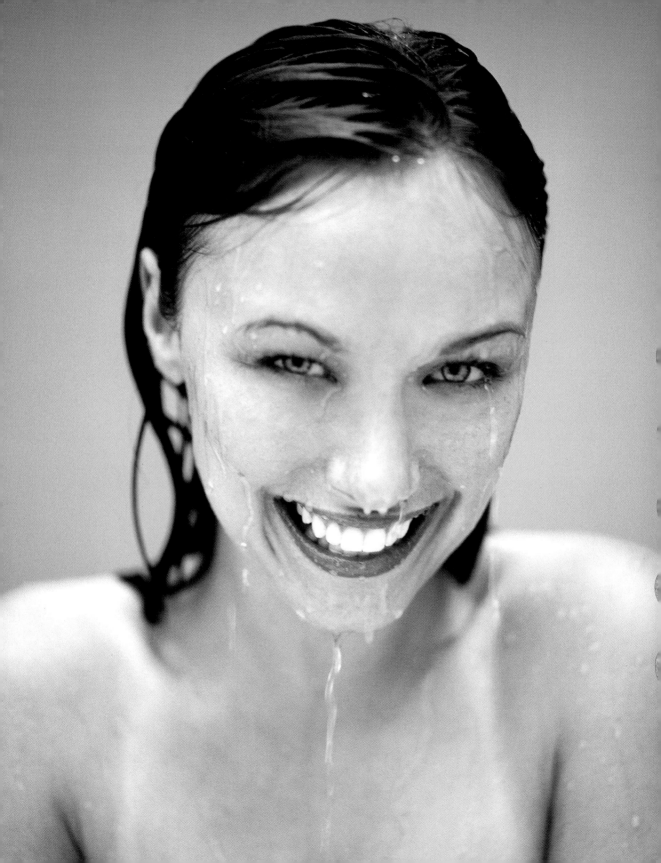

CHAPTER THREE

HYDRATION
WATER EVERYWHERE

FLUSHING THE SYSTEM

When we put a load of dirty dishes in the sink it's logical to rinse the dishes with hot water afterward, rinsing the sink at the same time. We're essentially flushing the system. The same applies to putting a load of vegetable peels into the garbage disposal. Water must be run through the pipes to flush the system. If not, bits of food are left to decay and things begin to smell bad. That's not dissimilar to why the body needs water in adequate supply. Without it nutrients would not be delivered to their final destination and toxins would not be carried away. With nothing to perform these essential tasks, the body seizes. It is possible to survive for weeks without food but possibly only one day without water. Since we humans are seventy percent water, we need to pay attention to drinking enough every day.

THE MIRACLE LIQUID

Water is a miracle liquid. It's true. Take a look at yourself. You are a mixture of water, protein and a myriad of molecules blended together to create the physical you. You are nothing short of a miracle. Two-thirds of you is water. Cells, bones and blood both hold water and float in it. Muscles are 75 percent water. According to **Alice Kavounas**, author of *Water Pure Therapy*, "You need water to enable your body to keep eliminating toxic substances, to produce digestive enzymes, maintain healthy skin, hair and organs, and to help your body absorb essential vitamins, minerals and natural sugars. Water also regulates your body temperature, cooling you down by evaporating through your skin."

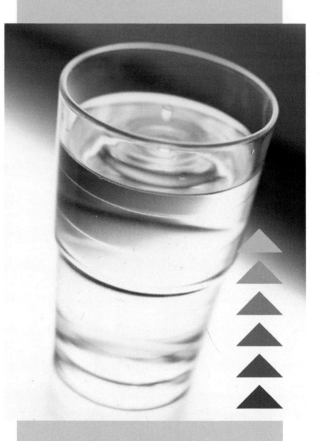

It is possible to survive for weeks without food but possibly only one day without water.

Even on a cold winter day your body will use and lose about two liters of water. Imagine how much greater that amount is on the hottest summer day. Athletes, active people and now you, on your Clean-Eating regimen, require much more than two liters of water every day.

HOW MUCH IS ENOUGH

But what's enough? Most physicians and health experts recommend drinking eight 8-ounce glasses of water per day. For some of you, drinking 64 ounces of water is a chore – and one that doesn't get done very well. For others drinking enough water is an obsession in which you carry your water with you wherever you go. Finding a bathroom then becomes a chore. Each of us is different – academic statement, I know! But because we're all unique what's enough water for one is not enough for another. One fact is true: water plays a critical role in regulating body temperature and metabolic rate. According to **Dr. Philip L. Goglia**, author of *Turn Up the Heat,* "The correct daily amount of water intake is approximately one ounce of water per pound of scale weight." Drinking less than this causes dehydration and even the least amount of dehydration slows metabolism and bodily function. "Without enough water, organs can't function as efficiently, so your metabolism slows to conserve energy," states **Molly Kimball**, a registered dietician at the Ochsner Clinic Foundation.

Are you well hydrated? To get the quick answer, check your urine color. If it's pale yellow or clear

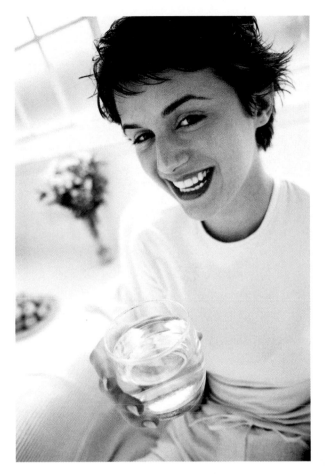

you're well hydrated. If your urine is deep yellow and murky you are not.

EAT CLEAN AND KEEP HYDRATED

This new Clean-Eating nutrition plan will help keep you hydrated, since fruits and vegetables are naturally juicy. Think melons, citrus fruits, cucumbers, tomatoes, celery, and lettuce. Part of the Clean-Eating strategy is to drink water with each of your six small meals.

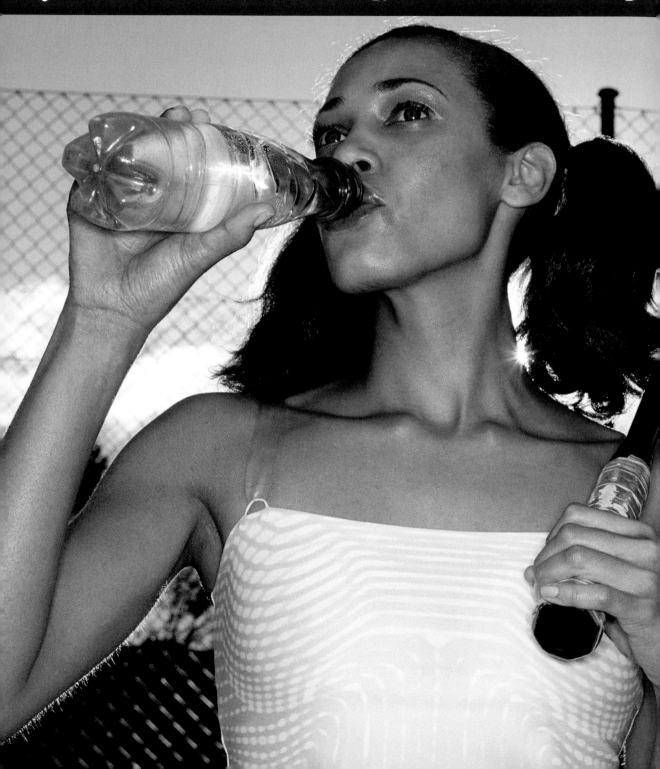

✳ Don't wait until you are thirsty

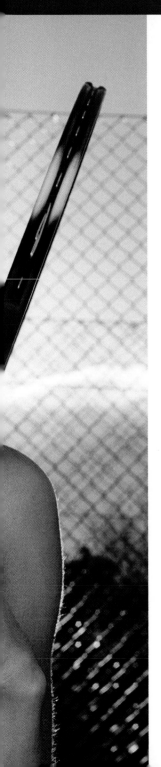

to drink water.

Get into this healthy hydrating habit without delay and you will immediately feel improved energy. On another note, starting your day by drinking two 8-ounce glasses of water (or 1/2 liter) before putting anything else in your mouth encourages lazy bowels to get moving.

I have a girlfriend whom I have known for more than 25 years. She only moved her bowels once a week, if she was lucky, for all of those 25 years. I had combated similar problems by Eating Clean, adding flax to my diet and drinking more water. So I told her about my success. She was happy, even elated to tell me that within weeks all systems were go every day, which is more like the norm. She lost 20 pounds of weight in the course of two months as well. All by drinking water and Eating Clean!

THIRSTY IS TOO LATE

Don't wait until you are thirsty to drink water. If you are thirsty it's already too late. Many of us have trouble deciding when we are thirsty. I know I am thirsty when I feel sluggish or tired, experience headaches (which I don't normally get unless I need water), have trouble concentrating or am constipated. When I work out I know I should hydrate myself so I do it throughout my workout and afterward. But if I'm just running around doing errands or sitting at my desk writing for long periods of time, I'm less tuned in to my thirst. A dry mouth and a flushed or tired feeling are all signs that I'm thirsty but I've clued in too late.

Thirst is a tricky phenomenon to understand. The feeling of thirst is governed by the hypothalamus in the brain. It reads salt levels in the body. When you are dehydrated, the salt concentration in your body rises. That triggers your thirst alarm. But by this time many of your vital organs are already severely deprived of water. That's why Clean Eating was the perfect answer for me. I rarely thought about drinking water when I was a frumpy housewife. I drank coffee; too much of it. I often felt lethargic and clammy. Did I mention I was frequently constipated? Come on, we have to talk about these things! Now that I schedule water drinking into my eating on a regular basis, I never feel as bad as I used to feel. Not only does Clean Eating drive you to eat correctly, it encourages you to hydrate yourself properly.

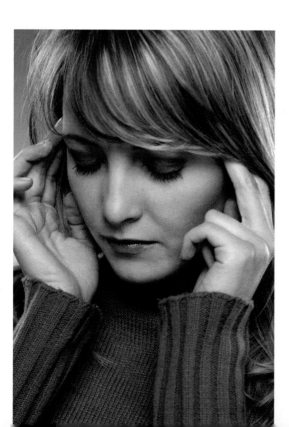

SIGNS OF DEHYDRATION

- Fatigue
- Lethargy
- Irritability
- Headache
- Blurred vision
- Flushed skin
- Lack of mental clarity
- Constipation
- Cystitis
- Back pain
- Excess weight
- High cholesterol
- Cellulite
- Water retention

MY WATER STRATEGY

I had to learn to drink adequate water. But like many of you, it was difficult to remind myself to do it. So I had to develop strategies to guarantee I would get two liters of water down every day.

HOW I DID IT!

I'm often on the go so I needed to be able to take enough water with me. In the beginning I would carry four ½-liter water bottles around and drink them throughout the day. Then I found it easier to fill a Nalgene bottle with fresh, UV-filtered water. Larger Nalgene containers hold one liter of water. I would either carry two with me or refill during the day. I'm a visual person so I found I was more successful at getting two liters of water down when I measured it out in advance.

DOES COFFEE OR TEA COUNT?

Both coffee and tea are diuretics, which means they take extra water with them when the body processes them through digestion and elimination. That's not good. Even worse, they take vital nutrients and minerals with them on the way out. Many health experts suggest giving up tea, coffee and wine for this reason. I will give up many things to Eat Clean but I refuse to give up coffee. I gave up the cream I used to drink in my coffee so I could spare myself those calories and the fat but I won't give up coffee. I drink it black and I do it early in the morning. One or two cups early on are acceptable. I take my vitamins at night so I don't pee them out with my coffee in the morning.

MY WATER INTAKE FOR THE DAY

6am	500 ml before breakfast and before anything else goes in my mouth
7am	500 ml with breakfast
10am	500 ml with mid-morning meal
1pm	500 ml with lunch
4pm	250 ml mid-afternoon meal (more if I need it)
6-9pm	250 ml with dinner 250 ml during workout 250 ml after workout

FEELING BETTER

I believe when you begin Eating Clean you will experience positive changes very soon, especially as you increase your water intake. I noticed my hair, skin and nails looked healthier. My facial skin became less textured with fine lines, and more radiant. The more I got used to the habit of drinking adequate water, the better I felt.

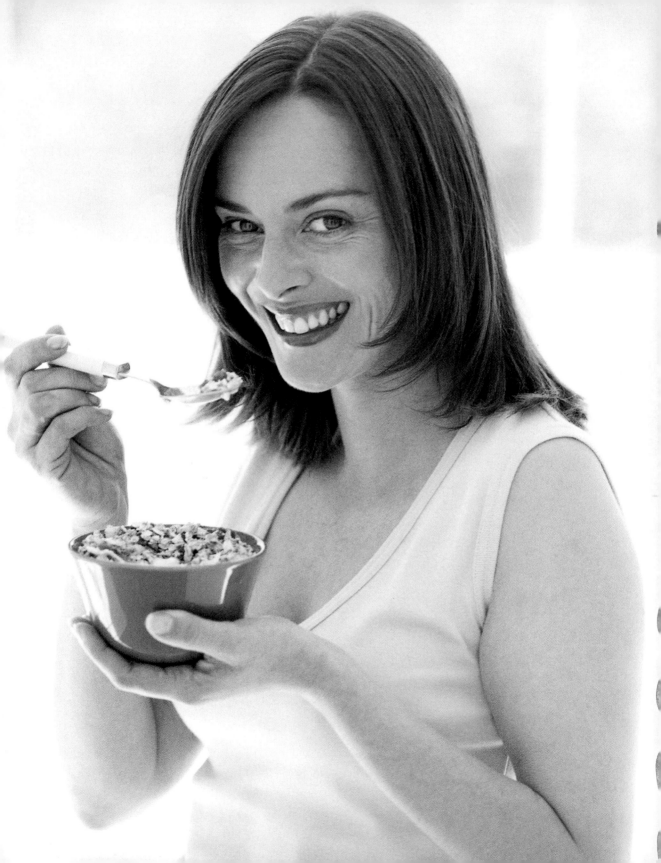

CHAPTER FOUR

BREAKFAST
A REALLY IMPORTANT MEAL

If you are serious about Clean Eating and making healthy changes in your life then you'll have to put down the doughnut and listen up. Study after study shows that if you start the day with a quality breakfast you'll tend to be leaner than those who skip this crucial meal. It's no wonder! If you are filling up with a bowl of hot oatmeal first thing in the morning you won't be tempted to scarf down unhealthy garbage when you are being attacked with hunger pangs later.

However, for many North Americans, eating breakfast is just one more thing to squeeze into a hectic morning. When most of us are already pressed for time there is a danger of trading a healthy breakfast for nothing at all, or for something sugary, greasy or fat laden at the drive-thru on the way to work. You and I might be able to rely on that poor technique to feed ourselves, but our children don't have the ability to pull up at the local coffee shop. When they leave home without breakfast they have no choice but to go hungry. There is no worse feeling

than that gnawing, empty burning at the bottom of your stomach. Even worse, starting your day without breakfast interferes with brain and physical function. Eating sugary, calorie-laden foods is of no use, either.

WAS THAT YOUR STOMACH GROWLING?

I'm sure you have noticed that when you are totally hungry the stomach makes noises – sometimes loud ones! Those growling sounds happen when the stomach walls squeeze together trying to digest and mix food that isn't there. After a long night without food, it is not unusual to hear the growling of a very empty stomach.

During the night the body takes much-needed time to repair itself from the day's activities. Tissue repair burns up plenty of fuel, and night is when all that repair takes place. However, throughout the night you are not taking in food or water, so you wake up dehydrated and hungry. That explains why your stomach is making so much noise. A night without eating leaves blood-sugar levels at their lowest. Blood sugar, or glucose, is the fuel the brain and body depend on for proper function. To offset this depleted state you need proper, Clean-Eating foods. You need breakfast!

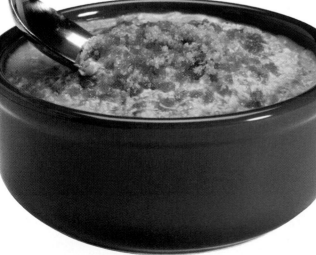

Just one cup of cooked oatmeal contains 8 grams of fiber, which accounts for almost a third of the recommended daily amount.

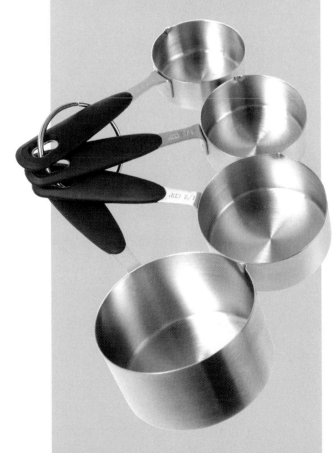

BREAK THE FAST WITH OATMEAL

When you wake up ravenous after a good night's rest the best thing you can do is "break your fast." The word "breakfast" implies just that. But before anything solid passes through your lips remember you are dehydrated too. Your cells are crying out for water. Drink two 8-ounce glasses of water so this essential liquid can get started on replenishing your thirsty cells.

No breakfast choice in the Clean-Eating plan includes sugary, calorie-laden cereals or pastries. The best solution to your breakfast growlies is oatmeal or other hot cooked cereals. Why? Because, as Grandma used to say, oatmeal is good for you and it sticks to your ribs. Oatmeal is so nutritious it is one of the first foods to be recognized by the Food and Drug Administration as having medical benefit. Oatmeal is loaded with soluble fiber, or plant fibers, helpful in controlling blood sugar and reducing blood cholesterol levels. The plentiful fiber in oatmeal also helps control weight loss or gain. Most North Americans don't consume enough fiber – the recommended daily amount is 25 to 30 grams a day. Just one cup of cooked oatmeal contains 8 grams of fiber, which accounts for almost 50 percent of the recommended daily amount.

A full tummy discourages you from snacking on sugar-laden or greasy junk throughout the day. A recent study of 3000 people showed that those who ate plenty of fiber each day, at least 25 grams, were less likely to gain weight. The results, published in the *Journal of the American Medical Association,* suggest that high-fiber diets keep weight gain at bay by reducing insulin secretions. Consuming plenty of fiber lowers blood sugar and insulin levels and reduces the incidence of cardiovascular disease.

Oat products such as oat bran and whole-oat flour also contain insoluble fiber, or "roughage." Unlike soluble fiber, insoluble fiber is not digested. Instead it moves through the digestive tract, cleaning it out and reducing the chances of getting certain types of cancer. The best sources of insoluble fiber include wheat bran, wheat-bran cereals, whole-grain breads and pastas, fruits, vegetables, nuts and seeds.

The American Dietetic Association supports these findings. The Association suggests that adults who eat breakfast have an easier time losing weight, while those who don't are 460 times more likely to gain weight. That is a significant reason to eat oatmeal, don't you think?

The best sources of insoluble fiber include wheat bran, wheat-bran cereals, whole-grain breads and pastas, fruits, vegetables, nuts and seeds.

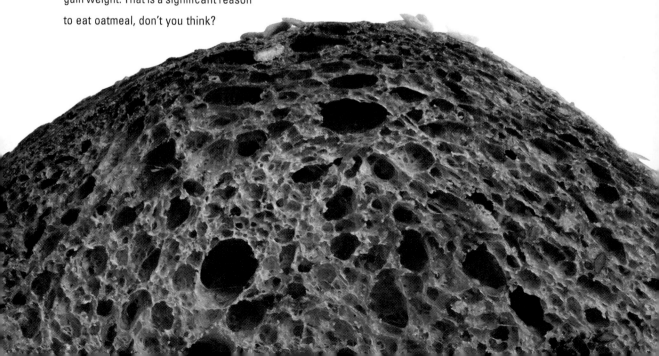

There is no better way to start your day than with a steaming bowl of oatmeal.

IT TAKES MORE THAN A BOWL OF OATMEAL

Oatmeal does not stand alone as a substantial breakfast. Clean Eating advocates eating a diet *low* in simple sugars, *low* in simple carbohydrates and *low* in saturated or trans fats. Imagine eating a bowl of oatmeal only to chase it with a platter of greasy sausages or bacon. YUCK!

If you have been following along with the principles of Clean Eating you know that you have to incorporate protein in your morning meal. While oatmeal has some plant protein it is usually not enough. But what are the Clean-Eating protein sources? Sausages and bacon are loaded with fat and nitrates, so they are off limits. Your cleanest protein option is egg whites or protein powder. Egg whites provide high-quality complete protein and contain amino acid combinations similar to those found in the human body. That makes them easier to digest and absorb. The egg is such an excellent protein source that it is actually the standard against which all others are measured. Egg whites are perfect for a Clean-Eating breakfast. Do consume egg whites only. The yolks contain a considerable amount of fat. It's all right to eat one yolk, but you should eat at least three or four egg whites alongside.

Egg whites can be eaten in many forms. They are highly versatile. Hardboiled eggs are easy to make for breakfast and convenient to pack into a lunch if there are a few left over. In fact they keep so well it's a good idea to prepare planned leftovers. Scrambled egg whites are delicious too, especially if you get creative and add vegetables and herbs. The possible combinations are endless. Adding vegetables to the egg whites fits in to the Clean-Eating principle of combining protein with complex carbohydrates.

One of my favorite egg-white combinations is served at the popular Firehouse Restaurant in Venice, California. The egg whites are scrambled with ground turkey, fresh cilantro, fresh tomato and spinach. Add a cup of steaming black coffee and a

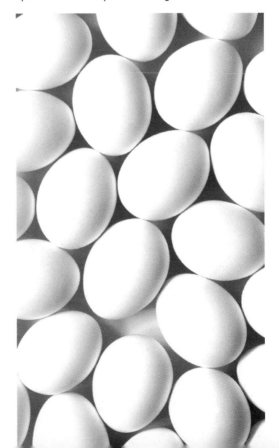

Adding **vegetables** to the **egg whites** fits with the **Clean-Eating** principle of combining **protein** with complex **carbohydrates.**

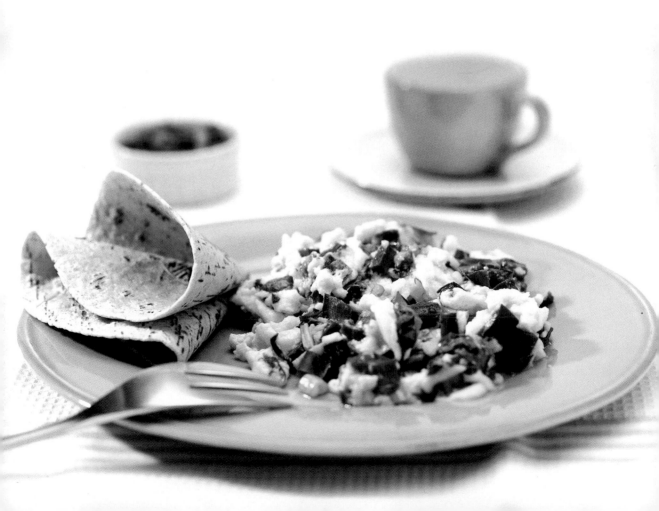

bowl of their delicious oatmeal and you're good to go for the morning. The plate is brimming with clean, lean protein piled so high it's a wonder anyone finishes it. Bodybuilders, fitness athletes and regular folk flock there to enjoy the Clean-Eating menu served all day long. I always have to laugh at the people who stand in line to order an egg-white omelet, watching over the chef to make sure he doesn't put any oil in the frying pan, but then asking for a load of cheese in the middle of the omelet. Regular cheese contains at least 50 percent fat! I very rarely have cheese in my omelet. If I must have it I use reduced-fat hard cheese or goat cheese, which is lower in fat.

Another way to add protein to the morning meal is to use protein powder. It can be mixed into your bowl of oatmeal or cereal or it can be used in a blender smoothie. Make sure to look for a high-quality protein powder that does not contain a lot of filler. I also check the label for added sugars. Many protein powders taste good and are creatively flavored with artificial sugars but you want to avoid these as much as you can. They are not ideal for Clean Eating. I also don't like artificial sweeteners because it is not clear whether they are safe and healthy. I avoid them at all costs.

GET FRUITY

Now let's add fruit to the breakfast mix. An easy way to incorporate one of the several suggested servings of fresh fruit into your daily intake is to toss fresh berries onto your cereal, hot or cold. Raspberries,

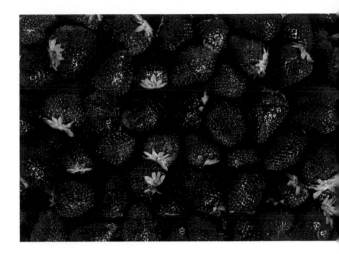

blackberries, strawberries, blueberries and all other berries are loaded with antioxidants and fiber.

Fiber, of course, is essential for many reasons already discussed in the section on oatmeal, but what are antioxidants for? These phytochemicals are powerful plant chemicals that absorb and neutralize free radicals. Free radicals are dangerous molecules I like to call "loose cannons." They are atoms or groups of atoms with unpaired electrons, formed when oxygen interacts with molecules. They are loose cannons because once they have formed a chain reaction of damage is launched. The biggest danger comes from the damage they do to the cells, especially DNA in the cell membrane. If a cell membrane has been attacked by a free radical it loses its ability to function properly and it may even die. Antioxidants help prevent the loose cannons from firing by mopping them up.

If you aren't interested in the chemistry lesson you will enjoy the flavor of berries, so why not toss a half-cup of mixed berries on top of your oatmeal? If you don't like berries on porridge or cereal, consider mixing up a bowl of fresh fruit salad with a combination of amazing fresh fruits including melons, kiwis, apples, pears, citrus fruits, peaches or whatever is in season. This can be eaten on the side for breakfast as well as later in the day when you get a snack attack.

STEPPING UP YOUR BREAKFAST NUTRITION

I never eat a bowl of cereal without adding a few special ingredients first. Flaxseed, bee pollen and wheat germ are my nutritional all stars. I love how they taste and how they make me feel. Both wheat germ and flaxseed are loaded with essential fibers while bee pollen contains an alphabet of vitamins, minerals and nutrients. It's like eating health in a bowl.

IN A RUSH?

I know what you are going to say. You are just too busy to even consider eating breakfast in the morning. Right? You may think this is the case but if you have a morning commute then you have time to eat breakfast. It is not ideal to eat while you are rushing around but if it is the only way then it must be so. Take along a container of premixed seeds and nuts, a piece of fruit like an apple or pear, a container of low-fat yogurt and you'll be better off than skipping breakfast altogether.

One of my favorite breakfast tricks I depend on, especially when I travel, includes preparing a container of pre-mixed dry oatmeal with flaxseed, bee pollen and wheat germ. I also add two scoops of protein powder and some raisins, dried cranberries or cherries. Then when I get to work or even to the airport I get a cup of hot water. I mix this into my "breakfast mixture" and voilà, breakfast!

Another of my favorite breakfast tricks is to set the breakfast table the night before. I like to do this because I insist on having meals as a family. North Americans are so time stressed these days that eating a meal as a family seems a luxury, but I believe it is the best way to teach healthy nutrition and keep a family together. So I set the table just before I go to bed. Colorful placemats and funky bowls make the table inviting. Cold cereal boxes can be set out along with glasses and silverware. If I am planning on having oatmeal for breakfast I set it up in the slow cooker or measure out the dry ingredients in advance and have them ready to go for the morning. Of course I always set up the coffee pot as well. Can't do without that!

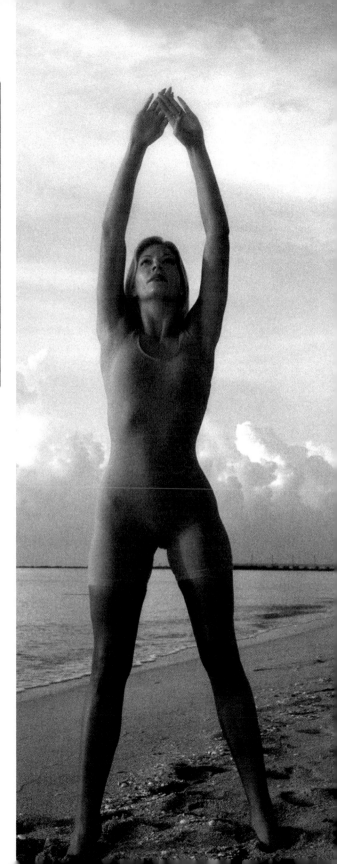

TIPS FOR WAKING UP
YOUR BODY

···❯ As soon as you wake up drink two 8-ounce glasses of water before putting anything else in your mouth.

···❯ Have a Clean-Eating breakfast of whole grains, fruit and vegetables, and lean protein.

···❯ Stick to natural, whole foods.

···❯ Avoid greasy processed meats and sugary, calorie-laden foods.

Drink two 8-ounce glasses of water so this essential liquid can get started on replenishing your thirsty cells.

POWERFUL PORRIDGE PREPARATIONS

WHOLE GRAIN	PREPARATION	COOKING TIME
Barley	1 part barley flakes to 2 parts water	Cook 45 minutes
Buckwheat/kasha	1 part buckwheat to 2 parts water	Cook 15 minutes
Millet	1 part millet to 2 parts water	Cook 30 minutes
Oatmeal	1 part oatmeal to 2 parts water	Cook 10 minutes
Wheat berries	1 part wheat berries to 4 parts water	Cook 1 to 1 ½ hours

SPICE IT UP

cinnamon,
nutmeg,
vanilla,
cloves,
allspice

FRUIT TOPPINGS

apples,
applesauce,
berries,
bananas,
melons,
pineapple,
citrus fruit,
raisins,
grapes,
peaches,
dried fruits

SWEET TOPPINGS

unsweetened
applesauce,
touch of agave
nectar

OTHER IDEAS

ground flaxseed,
bee pollen,
orange peel,
low-fat milk or
soy milk,
low-fat yogurt,
sesame seeds,
nuts,
sunflower seeds

CLEAN-EATING PORRIDGE

Here's a great way to start off your day with a Clean-Eating bowl of goodness. Make extra so it's ready for the next day or for a quick snack later in the day.

INGREDIENTS:

¼ cup each rolled oats, oat bran, rye flakes, barley flakes and ground flaxseed

2 cups water

1 tsp vanilla

¼ tsp each cinnamon and nutmeg

¼ cup slivered almonds

1 medium grated apple

INSTRUCTIONS:

Mix all ingredients in a heavy saucepan. Cover and place over moderate heat. When mixture comes to a rolling boil, reduce heat to low and continue to simmer for another 20 minutes, stirring continuously. When porridge is smooth and cooked through, remove from heat and serve.

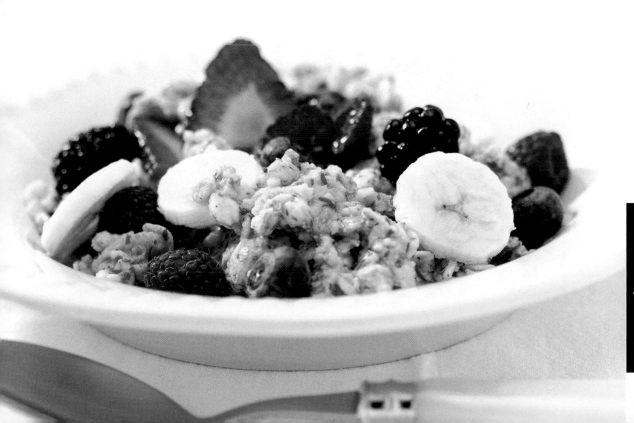

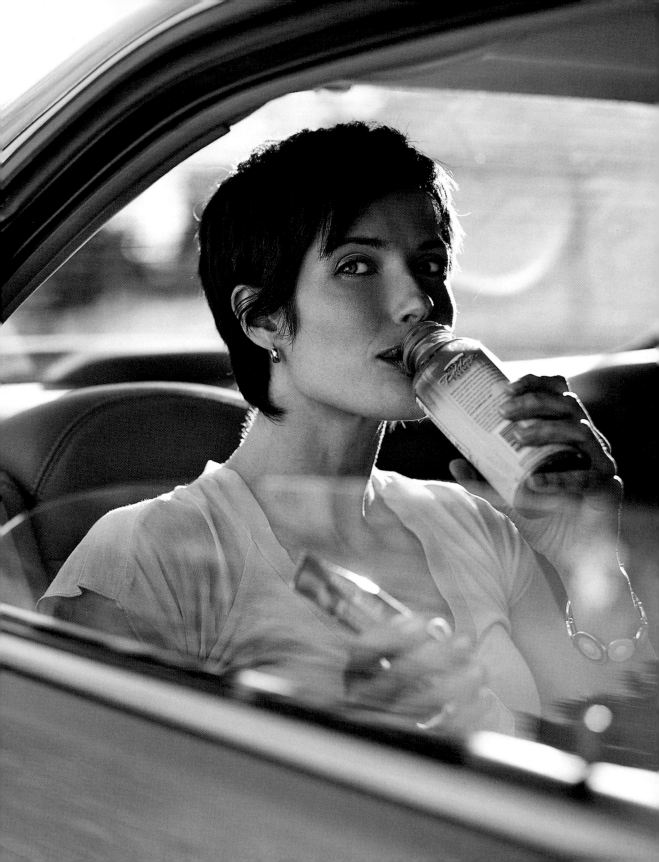

QUICK CLEAN-EATING BREAKFAST ALTERNATIVES

- Drinkable low-fat yogurt mixed with muesli

- Ezekiel bread with one tablespoon natural nut butter

- Hardboiled egg whites with dry brown toast

- Oatmeal with 2 scoops protein powder and handful raisins

- Scrambled egg whites on Ezekiel bread

- Protein smoothie with fruit

- Bowl of Ezekiel grain cereal with low-fat soy milk and berries

WHAT ARE EZEKIEL PRODUCTS?

The Biblical Ezekiel supposedly lived off of a hearty bread described in the Holy Scriptures as follows:

"Take also unto thee Wheat and Barley and Beans and Lentils and Millet and Spelt and put them in one vessel and make bread of it" – **Ezekiel 4:9.**

The bread sustained him while he lived in the desert for two years. It is a nutritionally complete food since it contains protein and complex carbohydrates in perfect balance.

Several companies today make Ezekiel bread and other live-grain products including cereals, muffins, bread, buns, wraps, bagels, energy bars, pita breads, cakes and pastas. Different from most breads available commercially, sprouted grain breads and products are made from freshly sprouted, certified organically grown live grains. None of these products contain flour.

References:
www.americandieteticassociation.com
www.obesitynetwork.ca
www.generalnutritiondirect.com
www.nal.usda.gov
www.whfoods.com
www.quakeroats.com
www.eatingwell.com

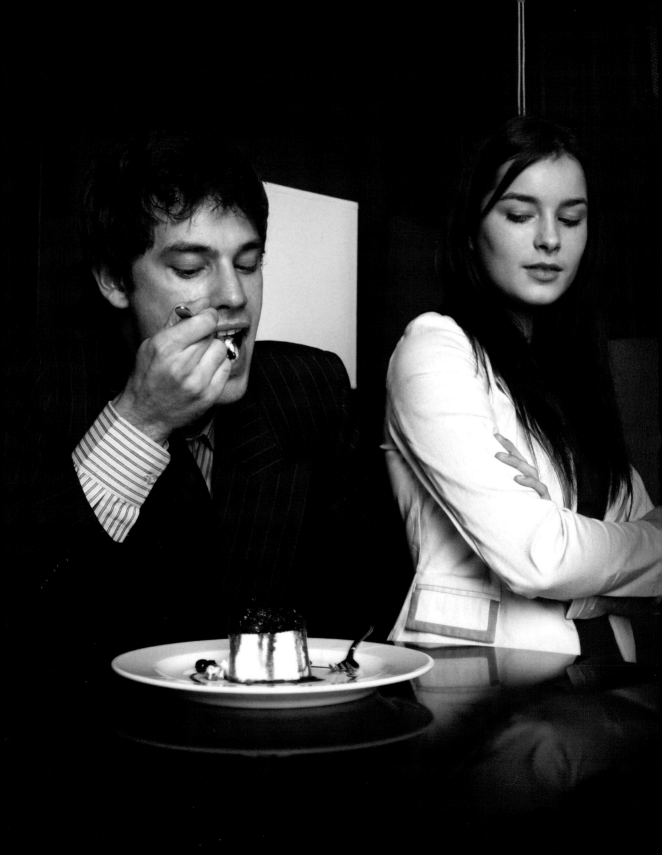

TURN YOUR BACK ON HAUTE CUISINE

GETTING STARTED

When I first discovered Clean Eating I confess I was uncertain that I would make the correct food choices. I had made the decision to Eat Clean and was so focused on doing it that I was scared to eat just anything. There's nothing worse than making the big decision to change your lifestyle, clean up your diet and think it is going to be the last time when you are confronted with the big problem … "What am I allowed to eat?" Digging into a pile of fries topped with gravy doesn't seem like such a good idea any more. But you're hungry. You've got to decide what's going down the hatch – you've gotta eat something! So what's it going to be for you?

NO MORE GUESSWORK

Knowing what to eat and when to eat it makes it simple to adopt the Clean Eating way of life. The lifestyle and habits accompanying it are what you need to get down pat. Once you do that, it's smooth sailing. Eating Clean takes the guesswork out of nourishing yourself and your loved ones.

2190 MEALS

Familiarizing yourself with the habits of Clean Eating will help you adopt this wonderful lifestyle. One of the most important habits is eating more food but of better quality. You have to eat every day – that's 365 days and at least six meals per day – or 2,190 meals over the course of a year. It doesn't hurt to figure out how to get it right.

Some of you may think eating twice as many meals per day as you normally eat is too much. However, you won't be eating six large meals, you'll be eating six smaller ones. You will spread your caloric intake out over your waking hours, at regular three-hour intervals. That's what I mean about eating more and making better choices.

Now about better quality foods. Eating more doesn't mean gorging on your old favorites. If chips and soda are the backbone of your diet today, you'll have to give them up. Don't wait another minute.

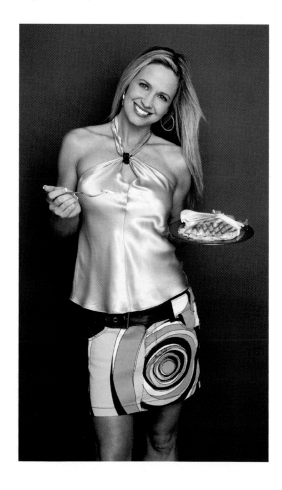

chapter five

FEEL HUNGRY FEEL FULL

Once you start Eating Clean you'll notice something very interesting. You'll learn how to feel normal fluctuations of hunger and satiation. The fuel you are eating on the Clean-Eating plan is so pure and of such high quality that it is burned cleanly and normally found accompanying your dinnertime steak are heavy on carbs and calories. By eating them at lunch you'll have a better chance of working them off, since you're busy and bed is several hours away. Eating a plate of mashed potatoes at 6:00pm with bedtime only three or four hours away just doesn't make sense. You'll never burn off the energy – and

One of the most important habits is eating more food but of better quality.

efficiently. That's why you'll feel yourself getting hungry fairly regularly at three-hour intervals. You will have to refuel because your body demands it. When you Eat Clean, your system is not working overtime trying to digest garbage that hangs around in your digestive tract like that ex-coworker you keep running into who feels the need to tell you how she *really* is every time you see her. These frequent smaller meals eaten at regular intervals of about two or three hours must contain complex carbohydrates and lean protein along with plenty of fresh water. That's the perfect formula for Clean-Eating nutrition.

DON'T GO BIG AT THE END!

It's also a good idea to throw out your old notions about sitting down to a big meal at the end of your day. Europeans always eat their heaviest meal at noon. What a brilliant idea! The starches and whole grains

there could be as many as 200 calories in a half-cup serving of mashed potatoes. Can you imagine how many there are in that big pile of mashed potatoes you love to eat? Hundreds! They won't disappear quickly while you're surfing channels in your easy chair.

MACRONUTRIENT RATIOS

→ **Protein:** 4 calories per gram

→ **Complex carbs:** 4 calories per gram

→ **Fat:** 9 calories per gram

MACRONUTRIENTS
DEFINED

SIMPLE CARBOHYDRATES are also known as sugars. They break down easily and tend to send blood-sugar levels out of control. Complex carbohydrates have a complex molecular structure that makes them more difficult to break down, and this helps control blood-sugar levels. In general you want to eat complex carbs and avoid simple carbs. Fruits are unusual in this respect. They are simple carbs, but they also contain plenty of fiber, which slows down their digestion, so you can eat moderate amounts of fruit. Make sure to pair your complex carbs with protein at every meal; again, to slow down digestion.

COMPLEX CARBOHYDRATES are high in fiber and improve digestion. They also stabilize blood-sugar levels, keep you satisfied after meals and provide loads of energy. Veggies, fruits, and whole grains are ALL complex carbohydrates. In fact, if the source of the food is a plant, and if the food is not a seed or nut, then it's a pretty good bet that it's a carb.

STARCHY COMPLEX CARBS

STARCHY COMPLEX CARBS FROM WHOLE GRAINS

*this is not an exhaustive list

+ Buckwheat
+ Multi-grain, buckwheat, Ezekiel, oat bran, and whole-meal spelt bread and wraps
+ Oat-bran cereal
+ Oatmeal
+ Quinoa**
+ Spelt
+ Sweet potatoes
+ Whole barley
+ Whole-wheat or brown-rice couscous
+ Whole-wheat, brown-rice or other whole-grain pasta
+ Wild, black or brown rice

STARCHY CARBS FROM VEGETABLE SOURCES

*this is not an exhaustive list

+ Bananas
+ Carrots
+ Potatoes
+ Radishes
+ Sweet potatoes
+ Yams
+ Garbanzo beans (aka chick peas)**
+ Kidney beans**
+ Lentils**
+ Navy beans**
+ Pinto beans**
+ Soybeans (aka edamame)**
+ Split Peas**

SERVINGS PER DAY

You should eat two to four servings of complex carbohydrates from whole grains or other starchy-carb sources each day. A proper portion of complex carbohydrates from grains or other starchy sources is measured by what can fit in one cupped hand.

**These are high-protein complex carbs and may be used as a protein source.

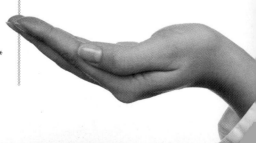

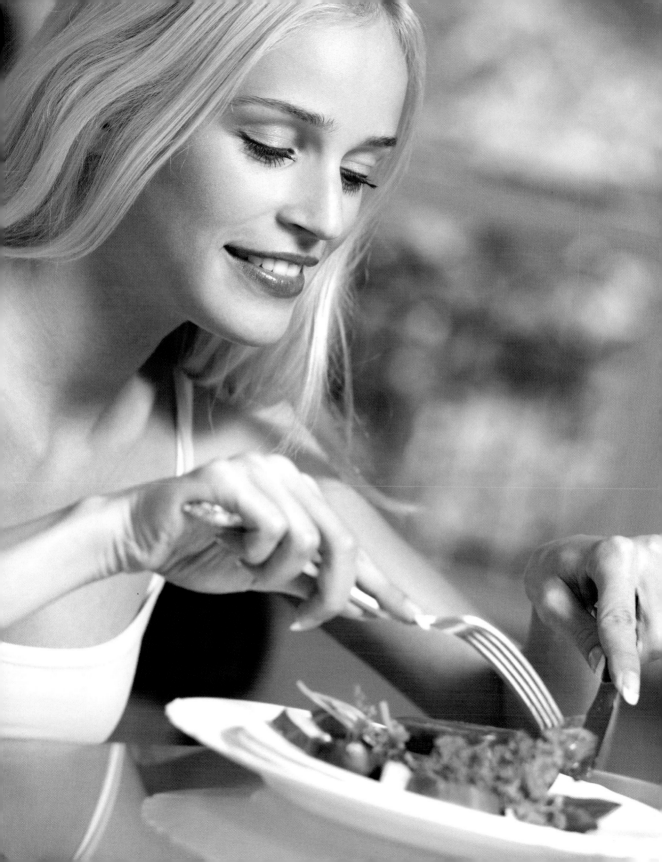

CARBS FROM FRUITS AND VEGETABLES

HIGH WATER-CONTENT COMPLEX CARBS

*this is not an exhaustive list

- Artichokes
- Asparagus
- Beet Greens
- Broccoli
- Brussels sprouts
- Cabbage
- Cauliflower
- Celery
- Cucumbers
- Eggplant
- Kale
- Lettuce
- Okra
- Onions
- Spinach
- Tomatoes
- Turnip Greens
- Watercress
- Zuccini

COMPLEX CARBOHYDRATES FROM FRUIT

*this is not an exhaustive list

- Apples
- Berries (strawberries, blueberries, raspberries, blackberries, etc.)
- Dried fruits in moderation
- Grapefruit
- Grapes
- Kiwi
- Lychee
- Mango
- Melon (cantaloupe, watermelon, honeydew)
- Oranges
- Papaya
- Passion Fruit
- Pears
- Plums
- Pomegranate

SERVINGS PER DAY

You should be eating from four to six servings of fresh produce a day. A proper portion of complex carbohydrates from fresh produce is measured by what can fit in two cupped hands. Remember if you are on the cooler-one plan to make sure most of your produce comes from leafy and fibrous greens.

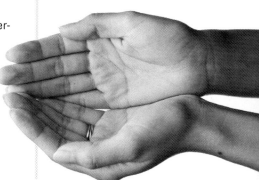

PROTEIN

Protein is primarily found in meat, poultry, fish and eggs, but is also found in dairy and to some degree in vegetable and grain sources. Tofu, chia seed (Salba), quinoa and hemp seed are complete proteins. Other plant sources must be eaten in combination in order to be complete. Animal protein is the most biologically available.

See page 25 for vegetarian protein options.

SERVINGS PER DAY

You should be eating five or six servings of protein a day, depending upon whether you have an evening meal. A proper portion of meat is measured by what can fit in the palm of one hand.

HEALTHY FATS

Healthy fats or essential fats are fatty acids that must be obtained from your diet because they cannot be produced by the body. Unsaturated fats are healthy, and those with a high level of omega 3 are best of all. These fats help your skin stay hydrated and lustrous, keep your cells working properly, help digestion and can also decrease inflammation in the body. And believe it or not, you need enough of these healthy fats in order to stay lean!

HEALTHY FATS

*this is not an exhaustive list

- ✦ Almonds
- ✦ Avocado oil
- ✦ Cashews
- ✦ Flax seed
- ✦ Hazelnut oil
- ✦ Olive oil
- ✦ Pecans
- ✦ Pumpkinseed oil
- ✦ Safflower oil
- ✦ Sunflower seeds
- ✦ Walnuts

SERVINGS PER DAY

Gram for gram, about 15 percent of your diet should come from healthy fats from fish, nuts, seeds, and healthy oils. If you are a calorie counter (which I don't advise), this works out to about 25 percent of your daily calories. Aim to include a few servings of these foods in your diet to ensure you are getting enough healthy oils.

tip When reading nutrition labels remember the word "hydrogenated" means trans fat, so stay away!

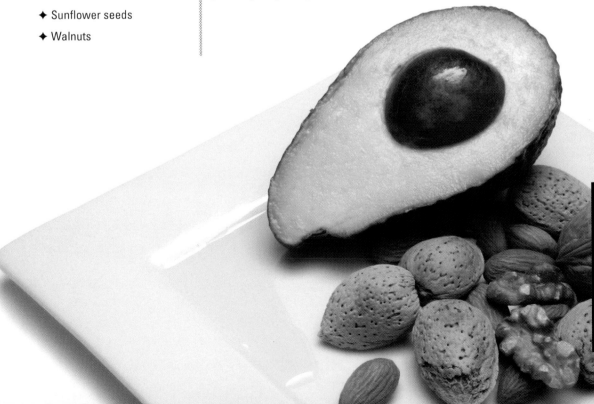

THE MAGIC OF PROTEIN AND COMPLEX CARBS

It is important to get the balance of nutrients absolutely right in each of your six meals. The real magic of Clean Eating occurs in the combination of foods eaten at each of these meals. *What is that balance?*

Lean protein + complex carbohydrates

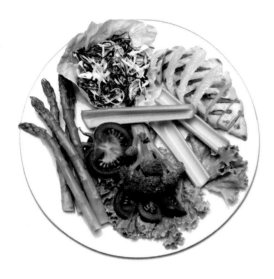

This ideal pair of food groups not only fuels the body with clean-burning fuel, but it causes a series of fat-burning reactions to occur. Imagine being able to eat and accomplish two things at once – feeding muscle tissue while burning stored fat! Remember, muscle is the only place in the body where fat is burned. The more muscle you have burning fat, the better your shape will be. In order to give your muscles a voracious appetite for fat you'll have to train them and nourish them properly.

PROTEIN PLUS COMPLEX CARBOHYDRATES

Protein is metabolized most efficiently in concert with complex carbohydrates. Empirical evidence shows this to be true. Your carbs need to be complex, not simple. The reason behind this is that complex carbs require more energy to be digested. So does protein. When both are present in the digestive system they work synergistically, one enhancing the other.

You will be interested to discover that eating this way makes you more aware of the body's cycle of hunger and satiety. The body consumes every last molecule of nutrients from clean foods with little left lounging about causing trouble.

SUGARS AND FATS— YOUR TROUBLE SPOTS

The sooner North Americans learn to recognize simple sugars and saturated and trans fats as Public Enemies Number One and Two in the same way they recognize germs in the bathroom as being vile, the sooner health will improve and waistlines will decrease. Ridiculous? Think about it! We sanitize, wash, and disinfect germs we can't see without hesitation but we consume, indulge, snack, wolf down and lick at sugars and fats without a second thought.

ENEMY FOODS

Sugars and fats are formidable enemies for the human body, eroding health and placing enormous strain on the endocrine system. In order to be successful with Clean Eating it's a good idea to know who your enemy is. Like the saying goes, *"Keep your friends close but keep your enemies closer."*

SUGAR

Popping up in the strangest of places – sliced deli meats, canned vegetables, soups – sugar is ubiquitous and ruinous to our health. The average teen now gets a whopping one-fifth of his or her daily calories from sugar and it is not even a food group! The average adult sugar consumption has increased by more than 30 percent in the last 20 years. Sugar's seductive sweetness wreaks havoc on the body.

FATS— THE FORBIDDEN FOOD

Health authorities would have us believe all saturated and bad fats come from meat. This couldn't be further from the truth. Many of the worst culprits hail from plant sources, including palm and palm kernel oil. Food corporations exist, well, to sell food. And to make as much profit as possible while doing so. They know that consumers like their food to have a certain "mouthfeel," and these fats are a cheap and easy, albeit unhealthful, way to accomplish this. Food corporations also add plenty of these and other dangerous "bad" fats to add flavor and prolong the

Sugar's seductive sweetness wreaks havoc on the body.

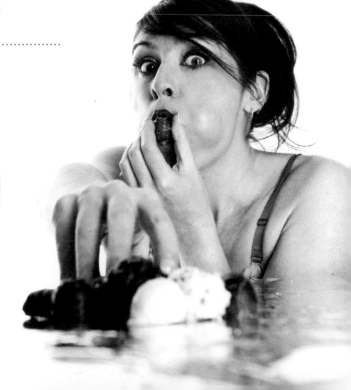

Try to keep your healthy fat intake to approximately **18%** of your daily food consumption.

shelf life of processed foods. In 1977 the amount of fat consumed by the average North American stood at 18 percent of total calories. In 1987 that number jumped to 28 percent and today the figure stands at a staggering 38 percent. The American Heart Association suggests that the total number of calories from fat should be kept to a lower percentage for optimal health. The ideal number of calories consumed daily from saturated and trans fats should be zero.

MEET FAT

There are three groups of dietary fats: **saturated, unsaturated** and **trans fats**. Saturated fats are mainly from animal sources. They are solid at room temperature. Think of great lumps of cheese, butter, tallow and lard. Saturated fats contain triglycerides, which are dangerous in the blood. Consuming too many saturated fats has been linked to an increased risk of several chronic diseases.

Trans fats are man made and completely unnatural to the body. However, they are found in many foods, since trans fats increase the shelf life of most processed food products. When you make the decision to Eat Clean, you also make the decision to avoid processed foods. By doing so you avoid consuming nasty trans fats.

Unsaturated fats include polyunsaturated and monounsaturated fats and are liquid at room temperature. Think of vegetable oils like flax, safflower, corn, olive,

sunflower and pumpkin. Unsaturated fats contain phospholipids – first-rate sources of essential fatty acids (EFAs). EFAs maintain cells and are necessary for hormone production, healthy brain function and a host of bodily functions. Consider eating just one tablespoon of ground flaxseed each day. Loaded with EFAs, flaxseed will boost your health in numerous ways, including increasing your fiber intake – great for lazy bowels. Flaxseed also makes you feel full longer, improves your hair, skin and nails, provides your body with loads of beneficial phytochemicals, which help to fight disease, and it has been proven in a recent study at the University of Toronto to reduce tumor size in breast cancer.

READ LABELS

To find out if what you are eating contains good or bad fats, check the nutrition label. All macronutrients are listed on the label according to new laws. Look for the "Total Fat" information, usually the third line on the label. Try to keep your healthy fat intake to approximately 18 percent of your daily food consumption. There will also be a number reflecting grams of saturated fat. This is the one to watch out for. If a product says it has 20 percent or more of saturated fat, don't bother with it. Less than 10 percent is better, and of course 0 percent is best.

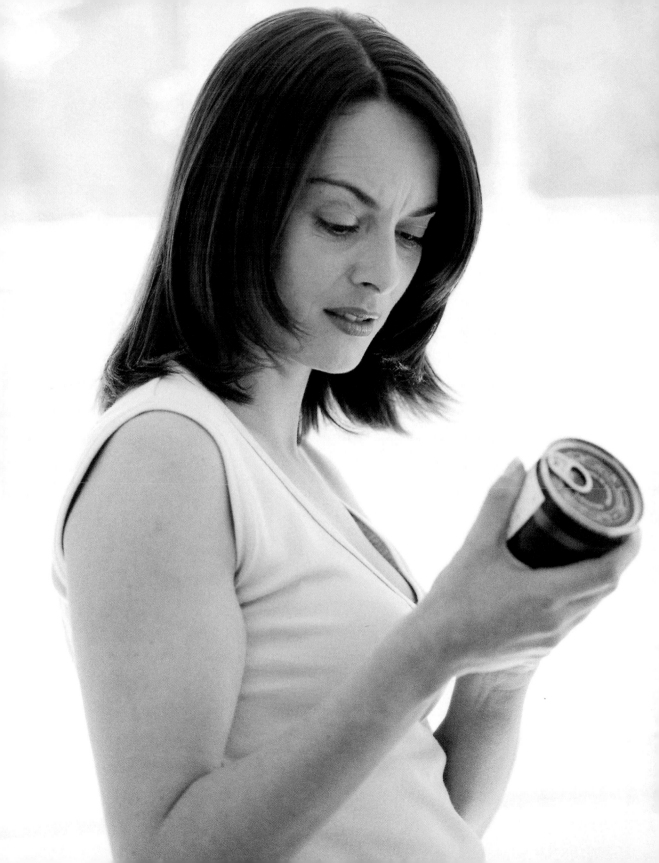

LET ME INTRODUCE YOU TO FAT

"**Fats** are lipid substances containing glycerol and fatty acids" according to *Larousse Gastronomique: The World's Greatest Cookery Encyclopedia.*

- **Fats** are in **solid** state at cooler temperatures.
- **Oils** are **liquid** at room temperature.

ANIMAL FATS

Some other terms used for **animal fat**:

- **Lard**, or **pork fat**, is used for cooking throughout Europe.
- **Beef suet** in England.
- **Sheep suet** or **sheep-tail fat** in eastern Asia.
- **Goose fat** in France.
- Scandinavian and Jewish cooks also use **goose fat**.
- **Calf fat** is used in forcemeats.
- **Smeun** used in North Africa.
- **Ghee** used in India.
- **au gras** = with fat.
- **au maigre** = no fat.

VEGETABLE FATS

Many people think that plants produce only unsaturated oils, but that is not the case. Most saturated vegetable fat comes from copra (or coconut), shea, or palm. Vegetable fats take the form of white, waxy rectangular blocks.

I EAT HEALTHY BUT I'M STILL FAT

I have had thousands of women e-mail me with the same question, **"Why am I still fat when I eat healthy?"** Since I know 80 percent of your physical appearance has to do with what goes in your mouth, the answer to these women is always the same. "You must tweak your diet and tighten up your eating habits." Then I ask them to journal and send me a few honest days worth of eating. That's when I set them straight.

The biggest traps I normally find are so-called "healthy" foods. Many foods disguised as healthy are higher in calories, fats and sugars than chips and soda. Low-fat snack foods may have reduced fat levels but are still loaded with sugar, so you're just trading one sin for another.

Often the women are eating yogurt, which is a healthy food, but they don't realize it is commonly full of sugar or other "bits and pieces" like fruit and chocolate. Peanut butter causes the same confusion, unless it's made from just peanuts. You would think peanut butter is healthy but when you have a look at the nutrition label you find it is loaded with sugar, and it has been hydrogenated – a euphemism for trans fat. Women often trip up on granola as well. Granola is healthy so they don't bother checking the nutrition label to see what's hiding in it. Granola can have more calories per serving than a bowl of Froot Loops.

There are plenty of places to get into trouble with packaged processed foods, so read the label carefully or, even better, Eat Clean!

ADDED SUGAR CONTENT OF FAMILIAR FOODS

Food	Added Sugar
Cooked cereals	0 tsp
Bread, 1 slice	0 tsp
Doughnut	2 tsp
Frosted or sugar-coated cereal	2-3 tsp
Cake, frosted, 1/16 or 8" cake	6 tsp
Double crust pie	5 tsp
Milk	0 tsp
Chocolate milk, 8 ounces	3 tsp
Chocolate shake, 10 ounces	9 tsp
Low-fat plain yogurt, 8 ounces	0 tsp
Low-fat fruited yogurt, 8 ounces	7 tsp
Frozen yogurt, 1/2 cup	3 tsp
Ice cream, 1/2 cup	3 tsp
Fresh fruit	0 tsp
Fruits, canned in juice, 1/2 cup	0 tsp
Fruits, canned in light syrup, 1/2 cup	2 tsp
Fruits, canned in heavy syrup, 1/2 cup	4 tsp
Sugar, jam, jelly, 1 tsp	1 tsp
Syrup and honey, 1 tablespoon	3 tsp
Cola, 12 ounces	7-9 tsp
Chocolate bar, 1 ounce	3 tsp
Sherbet, 1/2 cup	5 tsp

CARBOHYDRATE CONFUSION

Carbohydrates have earned a shoddy reputation in wake of recent fad diets. So infamous is the carbohydrate that it is universally blamed for North America's ungainly weight problem. What seemed like a good idea at the time – avoiding all carbohydrates – did work for a short while. But avoiding any food group will make a person lose weight. That's just mathematics. As people quickly realized, however, no-carb diets left them feeling awful, energy-depleted, and as fat as ever once they started eating carbs again.

It is folly to attempt to function on zero carbs. Have you ever tried it? It's difficult to manage even for a short while let alone an extended period of time. Your brain depends on carbohydrates for most of its energy, because carbs break down into glucose, which is readily accessible by your noggin. Experts advise eating about 55 to 60 percent of your daily total caloric intake from complex carbohydrates.

SLOW-BURNING FUEL

Complex carbohydrates from fruit, vegetables and whole grains are the best carbs for both brain and body while simple carbohydrates from refined sugars are not. Slow-burning complex carbs including oatmeal, brown rice, yams, and other vegetables and fruit, keep blood-sugar levels steady and keep you feeling full longer. Remember, when it comes to carbs go for the slow-burning fuel if you want staying power.

The importance of steady insulin levels is critical for balanced health and maintaining optimal weight. Insulin is a potent hormone for moderating blood-sugar levels, but also for storing fat. North Americans are deluged by hormone-imbalance diseases today.

Never before has a population faced the onslaught of obesity-related diseases we face today, many brought on by the overconsumption of fats and sugars. Sugar is everywhere. The can of soda in your hand contains seven to nine teaspoons of refined sugar. Eating a deli turkey sandwich? That's three grams of sugar per slice of turkey. Was that ketchup with your fries? More sugar! Candy virtually equals sugar. If it's not real sugar then it's fake sugar.

There are two different kinds of carbs and they are metabolized at different rates by the body: simple carbs burn quickly, complex carbs burn slowly. This impacts how food as fuel is burned in our body. At the same time it has a huge impact on appetite. Slow conversion, the ideal, keeps blood sugars steady so you don't experience that horrible, crashing, hit-the-wall feeling. As a bonus you don't get appetite swings, energy levels remain steady and you maintain a steady bodyweight. Complex carbs deliver all of these benefits. Where do we find complex carbohydrates? These are found in fresh fruits and vegetables as well as whole grains.

COMPARISON OF DIETARY FATS CHART

DIETARY FAT	FATTY ACID CONTENT NORMALIZED TO 100 PERCENT			
	Saturated Fat	Monounsaturated Fat	Polyunsaturated Fat	Linoleic Acid
Canola oil	7	61	11	21
Safflower oil	8	77	1	14
Flaxseed oil	9	16	57	18
Sunflower oil	12	16	1	71
Corn oil	13	29	1	57
Olive oil	15	75	1	9
Soybean oil	15	23	8	54
Peanut oil	19	48	*	33
Cottonseed oil	27	19	*	54
Lard	43	47	1	9
Palm oil	51	39	*	10
Butterfat	68	28	1	3
Coconut oil	91	7		2

*Trace

NO ICING ON THE CAKE!

Now that you are familiar with the enemy – sugars, saturated fats, and trans fats – keep them at bay and you will discover the dream physique that has been hiding under pounds of flab. Ridding your body of these enemy foods guarantees weight-loss success for a lifetime.

APPLES AND ORANGES

When Eve stole the apple from the Garden of Eden, sin notwithstanding, she had a brilliant idea. An apple is one of the best Clean-Eating foods you can eat, and its simple shape and robust color have come to represent healthy eating. It's a good idea to think of the apple as the snack food of choice on the Clean-Eating plan. The trick is to get you thinking the same way about a profusion of other clean foods so they too can make regular appearances on your plate. Enjoy the bounty of nutrients in beautiful green asparagus spears, crunchy snow peas, fragrant berries in every color, juicy red tomatoes and you'll soon get the idea – a refrigerator full of fresh fruits and vegetables in a rainbow of colors is like having suitable materials to build your perfect house. You don't want to build your dream home with junk and you wouldn't want to use junk to build your dream body either. This is how you should view foods as well – **you want the best to build the best.**

MENU PLANNING— A BLUEPRINT FOR SUCCESS

When building your dream home you wouldn't dive in without a plan would you? Similarly you need a plan to build your new body. Get into the habit of planning meals for each week so you know which materials you'll need to build them.

I am terrible at menu planning because I don't always know what I have in the house. I have two ways of combating this. My favorite tactic is to buy enough in-season fresh produce for a few days at a local market and build meals around those ingredients. For some reason I get very creative and inspired with piles of fresh fruit and vegetables on my kitchen counter. Four days is about the right amount of time to buy for since I feel one week is too long for fresh produce to keep. The other way I handle the menu is to stock a variety of Clean-Eating foods in my pantry so I'll never be caught short. I've included my Clean-Eating Checklist so you can provision your pantry properly.

Buy enough in-season fresh produce for a few days at a local market and build meals around those ingredients.

CLEAN-EATING CHECKLIST

THE BASICS

- [ ] **Herbs:** rosemary, basil, oregano, dill, mint, thyme, or other favorites
- [ ] **Spices:** red pepper flakes, cinnamon, nutmeg, cloves, allspice
- [ ] Sea salt
- [ ] Black pepper, peppercorns
- [ ] Balsamic vinegar
- [ ] Rice vinegar
- [ ] Low-sodium vegetable or chicken broth
- [ ] Low-sodium vegetable or chicken cubes
- [ ] Garlic powder
- [ ] Onion powder
- [ ] Lemon juice
- [ ] Lime juice
- [ ] Apple cider vinegar

STOCKING THE PANTRY

WHOLE GRAINS

- [ ] Brown rice
- [ ] Wheat germ
- [ ] Oatmeal
- [ ] Cream of Wheat
- [ ] Quinoa
- [ ] Bulgur
- [ ] Millet

NUTS/SEEDS

- [ ] Flaxseed
- [ ] Almonds, unsalted
- [ ] Cashews, unsalted
- [ ] Sunflower seeds, unsalted
- [ ] All-natural nut butters

CEREALS

- [ ] Shredded Wheat
- [ ] Ezekiel Cereals
- [ ] Some Mueslis (check ingredients)
- [ ] Ancient grains
- [ ] Brown rice cereal

DRIED FRUIT

- [ ] Apricots
- [ ] Raisins
- [ ] Dried apples
- [ ] Prunes
- [ ] Cranberries
- [ ] Cherries
- [ ] Figs
- [ ] Dates

CONDIMENTS

❑ Mustard

❑ Salsa

OILS

❑ Extra virgin olive oil

❑ Safflower oil

❑ Pumpkin oil

PANTRY

❑ Yams

❑ Sweet potatoes

❑ Potatoes

❑ Onions

❑ Garlic

❑ Squash

❑ Turnip

DRY GOODS

❑ Baking soda

❑ Whole-grain flours

❑ Baking powder

❑ Vanilla, best quality

❑ Sea salt

SUPPLEMENTS

❑ Bee pollen

❑ Protein powder

❑ Vitamins B, C, E

❑ Magnesium

❑ Calcium

❑ Omega-3 fatty acids

❑ Creatine

❑ MSM

❑ Daily multivitamin

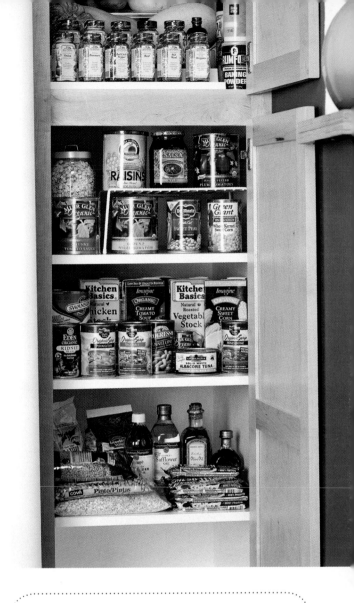

tip Stock a variety of **Clean-Eating foods** in your **pantry** so you'll never be caught **short.**

chapter five ■ 79

- ❏ Alfalfa
- ❏ Wheatgrass
- ❏ CoQ10

PANTRY

- ❏ Unsweetened applesauce
- ❏ White beans
- ❏ Chickpeas
- ❏ Lentils
- ❏ Kidney beans
- ❏ Bottled water, distilled and regular
- ❏ Canned tomatoes – crushed, whole and diced
- ❏ Tuna – water packed
- ❏ Salmon – water packed
- ❏ Low-fat soups
- ❏ Canned corn – low sodium
- ❏ Canned peas – low sodium
- ❏ Tomato paste
- ❏ Lemon juice
- ❏ Lime juice

FREEZER

- ❏ Whole-grain breads
- ❏ Whole-grain wraps
- ❏ Flash-frozen chicken breasts
- ❏ Pork tenderloin
- ❏ Fish
- ❏ Salmon
- ❏ Frozen berries
- ❏ Frozen vegetables

REFRIGERATOR

- ❏ Low-fat soy milk
- ❏ Skim milk with extra calcium
- ❏ Water
- ❏ Eggs
- ❏ Fresh berries – blueberries, raspberries, blackberries
- ❏ Cooked chicken breasts (always have six or more ready)
- ❏ Lemon juice
- ❏ Olive-oil based margarine
- ❏ Fresh fruits
- ❏ Fresh vegetables

TO TRANSPORT YOUR FOOD

- ❏ Small, portable soft-sided cooler
- ❏ Ice packs
- ❏ Re-sealable containers
- ❏ Plastic baggies
- ❏ Water bottles

A refrigerator full of fresh fruits and vegetables in a rainbow of colors is like the optimal materials to build your perfect house.

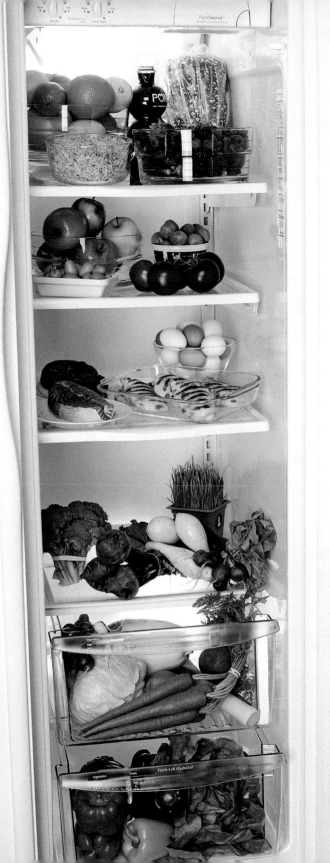
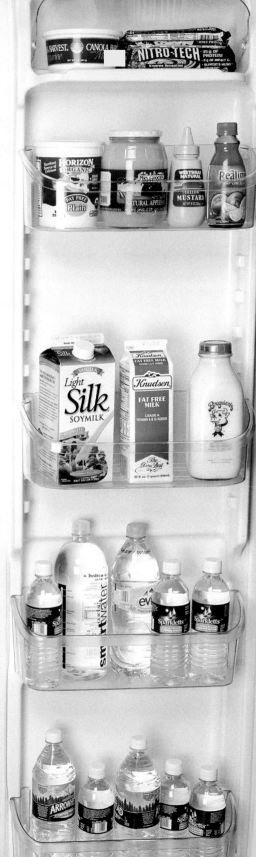

FEED ME! FEED ME!

Your most important meal is breakfast. Many of you think this is one meal that doesn't count so you don't bother eating it. Wrong! Skipping breakfast is the same as not putting gas in your car before a long road trip. How far do you think you can go on an empty tank? If you think you can outsmart your body and keep running on empty, you probably can for a while but you are robbing vital nutrients from organs in the process. Eventually the car runs out of gas and you are on the road to disaster, either sick, stuck or getting there. If you aren't providing your body with the nutrients it needs, it starts robbing your bones and muscles to get them. Not a positive scenario, is it? This can easily be avoided by doing something intelligent for yourself – it's called eating breakfast!

There is no better time than breakfast to set your nutritional standard for the day. You've not eaten for at least 10 hours. You're hungry and need refueling. A Clean-Eating breakfast doesn't include a trip to McDonald's, nor does it involve sticky pastries or sugary cereals. I've seen many people with a can of Coke in their hand at 6:00 am.

What a fabulous breakfast beverage! **Not!**

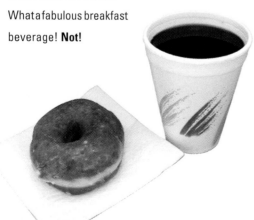

Instead fuel up on breakfast cereals based on whole grains including any combination of steel-cut oats, wheat germ, flaxseed, bulgur, barley, buckwheat groats, brown rice and quinoa. If you think you are Eating Clean with a bowl of muesli you might be wrong again. Store-bought granola and muesli mixes are usually loaded with sugar or sweeteners from honey, dried fruits, fruit juices, fructose and syrup. Make your own or look for no-sugar-added varieties. If you are interested in increasing your protein intake at breakfast, do so by adding egg whites to your hot cereal before cooking. Microwave and enjoy. It is an acquired taste, but many people love it. You also have the option of adding a scoop of protein powder to oatmeal if you don't like egg whites or if you want a change. The beauty of loading up on complex carbohydrates from whole grains like these is that you will feel full longer.

EVERY 2 TO 3 HOURS AFTERWARDS

It is 10:00 am, or three hours after you have last eaten. According to the Clean-Eating lifestyle you will need to eat. Don't take my word for it, listen to your stomach! You will certainly feel hungry by now and need to address that hunger. Don't pick up that loaded latté and Danish pastry. Your mid-morning snack should include the usual lean protein and complex carbohydrate. This magic combination will keep blood sugar and insulin levels steady, preventing you from crashing. Get complex carbohydrates from fresh fruit and vegetables and whole grains.

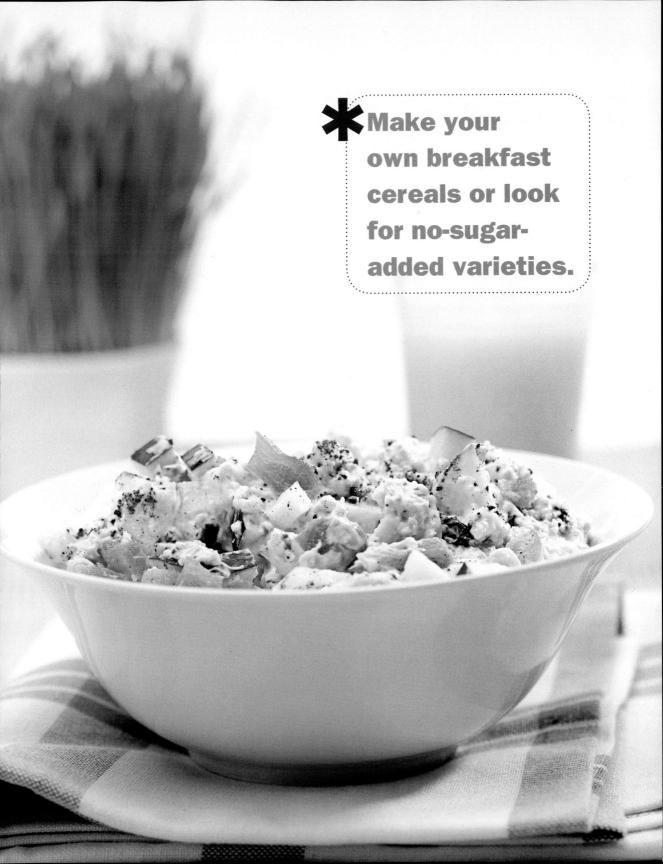

Make your own breakfast cereals or look for no-sugar-added varieties.

TEN UGLY FOODS

1 DONUTS: Even the humblest donut contains a whopping 490 calories and 30 grams of fat. Add a little sugar, jelly and whipped cream and you're looking at 600 calories and 35 grams of fat. The recommended caloric intake for a woman per day is only about 1800 calories. If several hundred of them are coming from one donut, which hardly satisfies the appetite, what are you going to eat for the rest of the day?

2 MARSHMALLOW FLUFF: This dandy stuff was the subject of heated debate recently as one mother tried to remove it from her child's school-cafeteria menu. One teaspoon holds 60 calories, but kids load much more than a teaspoon of the stuff on their sandwiches. This white poison contains nothing but junk! There isn't one speck of nutritional value to be found here. Made with corn syrup and gelatin, Fluff is similar to marshmallows, or chemical puffs, as I like to call them.

3 COLAS, SODAS, CARBONATED BEVERAGES: The average carbonated beverage contains approximately seven to nine teaspoons of refined sugar. That's a load of sugar! Most of us don't even realize we are taking in that much sugar while drinking a favorite carbonated beverage. Even fake sweeteners like aspartame or Splenda®, which are added

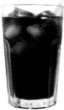

to diet sodas, may be detrimental to health. Sodas contain harmful chemicals and preservatives, none of which contribute to your health. North America's obsession with sodas is relentless. I have even seen young mothers feeding infants Orange Crush out of a bottle. What chance do these kids have? Better to quench your thirst with fresh water.

4 BACON, DELI MEATS AND PROCESSED MEATS:
Many North Americans could not conceive of a breakfast without bacon or sausage, a baseball game without a hot dog or a sandwich without sliced deli meats. I'm convinced if you knew what I know you wouldn't touch the

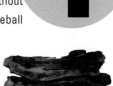

stuff again. What do you think hot dogs are made of? Consider fat content for a start. The average sausage contains 10 grams. A slice of bologna has 7 grams of fat, which is the same amount as a hot dog. Research shows a diet high in animal fats is linked to an increased risk of heart disease. Most processed meats contain a chemical soup of nitrates, nitrites, sugar, sodium and preservatives. Many of these are implicated as the culprits in disease, particularly cancer.

5 SUGAR-LOADED BREAKFAST CEREALS:
It always takes me a few minutes to negotiate the breakfast cereal aisle. I gaze up and down the length of it and think about the staggering array of boxed cereal available. Sooner or later a mother and her kids will come along. The choice of cereal is usually always made by the pushy kid. "But Mom, I don't like oatmeal. I want Captain Crunch." No doubt because of the sugar content. Strangely,

many folks add even more refined sugar to their bowl of cereal. Most cereals also contain a hefty dose of trans fats.

FRUIT JUICES AND FAKE FRUIT DRINKS: It's not hard to guess why these are bad choices. Fake fruit drinks are loaded with sugar. The same is true of fruit juice. Think of an orange. It comes wrapped in a neat serving size easily accommodated by the body. Plus it comes with lots of fiber. Now consider a glass of fresh-squeezed orange juice. Believe it or not, the amount of sugar in a 12-ounce glass of fresh squeezed orange juice totals 36 grams of carbohydrate, most of it from fructose, which is a simple sugar. This amount of carbs will push your insulin levels through the roof. There's far too much sugar at one gulp for the body to handle. Fake fruit drinks are even worse, since they are loaded with refined sugar or chemical sweeteners and food coloring. Drink fresh water to quench your thirst.

WHY DO YOU THINK THEY CALL IT JUNK FOOD? Potato chips, buttered popcorn, deep-fried snacks, Doritos – the North American species of couch potato loves these nibbles. Unfortunately such foods carry an unwelcome load of empty calories, trans and saturated fats and sodium. You can hardly call such products food. Avoid these at all costs. If you absolutely can't resist, at least measure one cup of chips and call that your limit instead of downing the entire bag.

CANDY, CANDY FLOSS, COTTON CANDY: Maybe I should just repeat myself. None of these treats qualifies as a food group since they don't contain any nutritional value whatsoever. They are calorie-dense, sugar-loaded, health-destroying time bombs. On top of that, artificial food coloring is used to make these so-called treats more appealing. Are there any redeeming qualities to this junk? Yes, you can use candy floss as emergency glue if you have nothing else available.

FRENCH FRIES: The "French" give fries their name. Belgians and Dutch insist on mayonnaise with their "patat" and North Americans douse them in ketchup. Another popular variation called poutine smothers the fries with melted cheese and gravy. No matter how you like your fries, any variation guarantees a heart attack or stroke along with a big fat belly. Cooked in enormous vats of (usually hydrogenated) oil that has been heated and reheated several times more, fries deliver unhealthy saturated and trans fats along with a side order of free radicals.

TWINKIES: The Blue Man Group pokes fun at how disgusting Twinkies are. It's even joked that Twinkies are made with so many preservatives they do not decompose in garbage dumps. During the '60s when the fear of being bombed was high, Twinkies were the item most purchased to stockpile in the bomb shelters because they "stay fresh forever." Just imagine what kind of chemicals these sponge cake "treats" have been doused with. If they don't decompose in a dump, what do you think happens to them in your body?

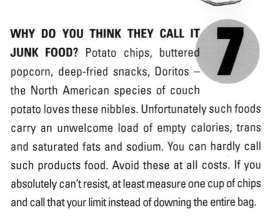

SHOPPING CLEAN

You have made a significant decision to change your current dismal nutrition into Clean Eating. It's beginning to get you excited. Very excited! You will discover a new slim physique, improved health and an abundance of energy, things you may not have experienced ever before reading this book. You can hardly wait to get started, but when you open your cupboards you are faced with the evidence of your previous bad habits. Time for a little spring-cleaning. You'll have to make room for the exceptional fat-burning clean foods you will be eating from now on. It's time to clear out the junk hiding in your kitchen, cupboards, fridge and pantry. If you don't you'll have trouble avoiding temptation in future.

So be honest and ruthless. Toss it all! Cookies, chips, Tostitos, Doritos, crackers, chocolate bars, sugary cereals, doughnuts, pastries, cake mixes and any other hidden goodies. According to **David L. Katz, MD**, author of *The Way to Eat,* "If a product is labeled 'reduced fat' you can generally be sure it's not low in fat, or it would say so! So-called healthy reduced-fat products are often still high in fat, they just have less than the standard version of the particular product." Beware of those foods! Even the chocolate, icing and baking supplies are off limits!

Don't want to make a list? Here's my list showing a cartful of excellent Clean-Eating shopping tips to guarantee physique success. Don't forget about your secret stash of beer or Grey Goose vodka. Alcohol is just another form of sugar. Having anything other than a bottle or two of dry red or white wine around to enjoy occasionally isn't going to help you find your tight new body.

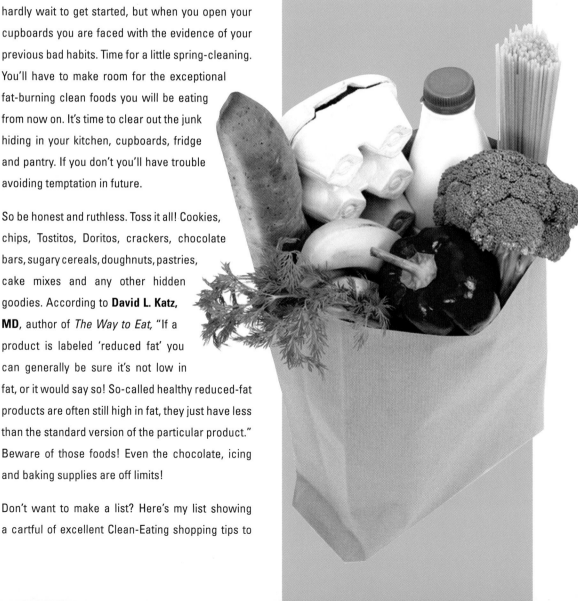

CLEAN EATING – SHOPPING CLEAN

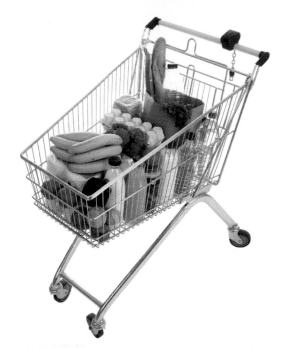

···⟩ **Create a menu** for the entire week using recipes you wish to try and shop from that list. Don't throw in unnecessary extras.

···⟩ **Eat before you go.** It is a proven fact you will overbuy and purchase foods you wouldn't ordinarily when shopping on an empty stomach.

···⟩ **Perimeter shop.** Shop the outside aisles of the grocery store first. This way you will hit the fresh produce, dairy and butcher sections before entering the packaged goods aisles, which are always at the center of the store. I usually have so much in my cart by then I don't have room for foods I should avoid anyway.

···⟩ **Shop solo.** You can get in and get out quickly and no one will bug you for a candy bar at the checkout.

···⟩ **Stick to your list.** Don't be tempted to buy extras just because they look interesting or are on sale.

···⟩ **Look for and avoid hidden sugars** including corn syrup, dextrose, fructose, glucose, gluco-fructose, honey, molasses, maple syrup, maltose, sucrose and artificial sweeteners. Nutrition labels list them all.

···⟩ **Read labels.** The nutrition label will also list total grams of fat per serving along with amounts of saturated fat and cholesterol. Watch for and avoid palm and palm kernel oil, shortening, butter, chocolate, milk chocolate, cocoa butter, egg and egg yolk solids, lard, tallow, suet, whole-milk solids, glycerol esters, and mono- or diglycerides. None of these are Clean-Eating options.

···⟩ **Avoid man-made trans fats and saturated fats at all cost!** According to **Lee Labrada**, author of *The Lean Body Promise,* trans fats "are the worst artery-clogging, cancer-causing substance you can put in your body." He's right.

···⟩ **Always look for the highest fiber content products,** especially in breads and cereals.

···⟩ **Be aware of "health" foods posing as healthy foods.** These products can contain more hidden evils than the original.

SHOPPING FOR PROTEIN

Clean Eating revolves around building a layer of fat-burning muscle, which is the engine that drives your metabolism and resultant weight loss. To have plenty of lean muscle you must train it and feed it. Feeding it means giving it lean protein. Not all high-quality protein comes from animals. When Eating Clean, replace animal protein with vegetable protein at least three or four times per week. Where does healthy vegetable protein come from? Beans! Don't laugh. Beans may be the musical fruit but they sing a different tune with their low-fat, high-quality protein

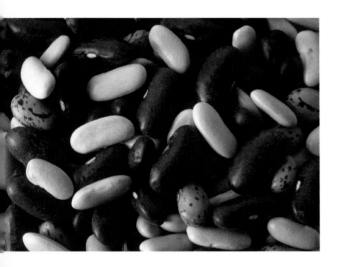

content. Try legumes, soybeans, chickpeas, lentils, all manner of white beans, black beans, kidney beans, black-eyed peas, pinto, fava, Lima and Romano beans. Keep an open mind for protein from quinoa and tofu. These options are less expensive than meat and taste yummy.

Everybody knows what ground beef is. It turns up in anything from chili to soup. Most ground beef isn't lean enough for Clean Eating but there are low-fat alternatives. There are several delicious varieties of ground meats including bison, buffalo, turkey and chicken that are easily substituted for fattier ground beef. Just read the label to make sure you aren't getting fat from skin or other excess fat in your mix. One hundred percent ground meat containing no skin or fat. Unsure? Have your butcher grind lean cuts of meat so you know for sure there is no extra fat. If you have the option to buy meat in portion sizes, do so. Look for 5- to 6-ounce servings, since this is the amount recommended for each Clean-Eating meal.

Buy "family packs" of meats, since buying in bulk makes it cheaper. They are a time saver too, because instead of buying and grilling one or two breasts of chicken you can grill several and have planned leftovers.

Turkey breast, chicken breast, pork tenderloin, beef tenderloin, buffalo and bison are the leanest cuts of meat. If you like venison or caribou, they too are excellent sources of lean meat.

Salmon, halibut, snapper, tilapia, cod, mackerel, water-packed tuna and sole are super sources of lean fish protein. Protein from fish is easily digestible. Also, fish contains essential omega-3 fatty acids. Shrimp and scallops are also good sources of protein and omega-3 fatty acids but tend to be higher in cholesterol. Eat these sparingly.

Eggs, the perfect source of complete protein, are versatile and inexpensive. If you consider the whole package, there is one slight flaw. Egg yolks contain cholesterol so keep your consumption to two egg yolks per week. Otherwise egg whites can be eaten every day in countless versatile ways.

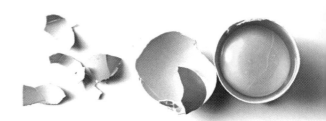

TRY THESE SUBSTITUTIONS
INSTEAD OF YOUR CURRENT FOODS

TOSS IT!	SWITCH IT!
Ground beef	Ground chicken, turkey, bison or buffalo
Bacon, back bacon, fatty pork, sausage	Pork tenderloin
Pastry, cake, cookies, candy	Fresh fruits, non-fat, unsweetened yogurt
Egg yolks	Egg whites
Chicken wings, ribs, hot dogs	Turkey or chicken breast
Whole milk, cream, half and half	Skim milk, low-fat soy milk
Cheese, cheese products	Low-fat cheese, cottage cheese, goat cheese
Full-fat yogurt, sweetened yogurts	Low or non-fat, plain yogurt
Cream soups, chowder, gravy	Clear soups, broth-based soups, broth
Chips, cheesies, nachos, crackers	Unsalted nuts, unsalted air-popped popcorn
Processed deli meats	Sliced chicken or turkey breast
Breads	Flatbread, pita, wrap, Ezekiel bread
Sugar-loaded cereals	Muesli, whole grains, shredded wheat
Cooking oils, lard, butter	Unsaturated oils
Dressings	Lemon juice, balsamic vinegar
White rice	Brown, black or mahogany rice

GOTTA DO THE GROCERIES

Grocery shopping often seems like a chore. And for most of us it is. But I enjoy doing my groceries. I like it because I am acutely interested in eating well now that I Eat Clean. I have to shop for a family that ranges in size from five to ten people, depending on who's home that week. Whatever I throw into my grocery cart ultimately ends up on the family dinner table so I enjoy making healthy choices right at the source in the grocery store.

Before I go shopping I usually have spent some time preparing a menu so I already know what meals I will be creating. The ingredient/shopping list is in my hand and I stick to it pretty closely. Of course there is the odd time I'll stray but that's because the fresh fish looks totally amazing or local produce is in season and it's too fresh and inexpensive to pass up – not because I'm starving and the Oreos are calling me.

Where I enjoy shopping most is in the produce section. I start my grocery shopping here, always. It's a habit I learned as a young child when I accompanied my mother on her grocery shopping expeditions. In the same way she fussed over making the best fruit and vegetable selections, I trouble myself over selecting the freshest-looking produce.

> **Choose a variety of produce colors— choose a rainbow of color.**

Choose a variety of produce colors – choose a rainbow of color. I have seen many shopping carts with nothing more than a few carrots and potatoes in them. To get the best array of vitamins, minerals, fiber and phytochemicals, choose produce in every color. Apples in any color possess flavonoids. Broccoli and its cousins contain isothiocyanates. Berries have lignans. Carrots, sweet potatoes, mangoes and apricots possess carotenoids. These are all potent antioxidants. Green leafy vegetables are important for fiber and for alkalizing the blood. Buy the freshest produce possible.

I always enjoy selecting the healthiest foods possible for my family and me. I also know that when I do the grocery shopping I don't buy junk. I leave it at the grocery store. If I bring it home everyone will be tempted to eat it and that's where the trouble begins.

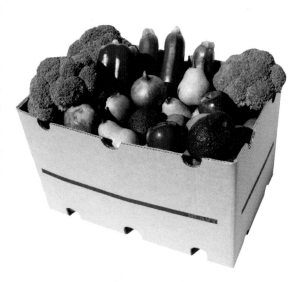

As you make your way to the checkout there may be more temptation greeting you. I've never seen a checkout loaded with fresh fruit or vegetables. While waiting in line you normally see candy bars, chips and soda, along with weight-loss magazines promising fad diets. You might be tempted to think, "What's one chocolate bar?" Forget it! Leave the chocolate bar where it is and ignore the trendy fad diets. You're Eating Clean now.

CLEAN-EATING FOOD PREP

Welcome home! It's time to put your groceries away and have a cup of green tea. Right, now load up your cupboards and refrigerator. When your refrigerator and cabinets are bursting with fresh produce, whole grains and an array of Clean-Eating foods, you'll be turning out delicious dishes with no trouble. Is it time for a grilled chicken breast wrap yet?

GETTING STARTED

Every craftsman knows the right tools make the job 100 percent easier. Stock up on basic kitchen necessities since the correct tools ensure Clean-

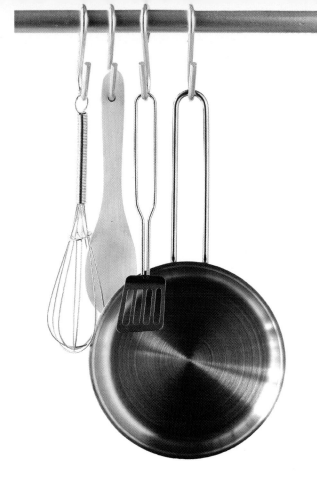

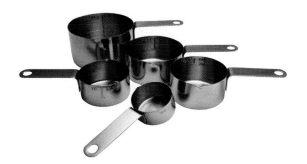

Eating success. Nonstick bakeware, including loaf pans, cookie sheets, casserole dishes and baking dishes are inexpensive and ideal for cooking many clean foods. They eliminate the need for greasy oils. One of my favorites is a nonstick grill pan with ridges on it, just like a grill. You don't need cooking spray or oil to cook meat since the nonstick surface prevents food from sticking. Lean chicken breasts done in the grill pan taste great and are practically fat free. You will need non-metal utensils and scrubbers for these pans since metal scrubbers will scratch and ruin the surface. Another wonderful tool for baking is a Silpat sheet. These are made of silicon and let you bake without requiring grease, spray, oil or paper liners.

A good blender makes the creation of smoothies or protein shakes a breeze. You may also want a small hand-held blender so you can blend soups right in the pan. Food processors and mini choppers save a lot of prep time in the kitchen, especially when it comes to chopping fruits and vegetables.

My Clean-Eating kitchen includes glass mixing bowls and measuring cups, a Dutch oven, nylon cutting board, microwave, storage containers, a rice cooker, crock pot, a quality set of knives and a quality set of pots and pans. I also like to use a clay baker for roasting chicken and turkey. Delicious!

PREPARING CLEAN-EATING MEATS

All visible fat should be trimmed from meat before cooking, including skin. It's best not to purchase fatty cuts of meat in the first place. Don't bother with gravy, most contain too much fat. Use low-sodium beef, chicken or vegetable broth instead. If you want

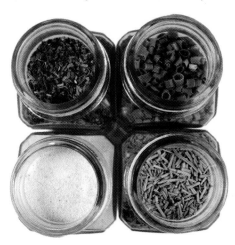

to add moistness to meats, consider using salsas as a side dish. They are wonderful mixtures of finely chopped fruits, vegetables and herbs that add flavor, texture and moistness to most foods.

Avoid crispy batters, crumb toppings or other meat coatings. The same applies to bread stuffing. Substitute whole grains, including brown rice or bulgur, for stuffing instead. Use herbs, spices and marinades to flavor meats. After you have prepared homemade soups, stews or chili, place the finished product in the refrigerator overnight. Any remaining fat will rise to the surface and congeal, making it easy to skim off the top before serving.

VEGETABLES, PASTA & WHOLE GRAINS

Beautiful, fresh vegetables are the ideal food to fill up your tummy. They come with a complete alphabet of nutrients and complex carbohydrates that are best enjoyed raw. So don't fall into the rut of cooking vegetables when you can munch them raw or lightly steamed.

After you've stocked your kitchen, spend a few minutes washing and cutting your goodies. Then they'll be ready for your appetite. Vegetables should be lightly steamed, stir-fried, roasted or par-boiled. Grilled vegetables, too, have a wonderful taste.

Instead of rich cream sauces try herbs, tomato sauce or other puréed vegetables. The possibilities are limitless. Look on page 242 for my Tomato and

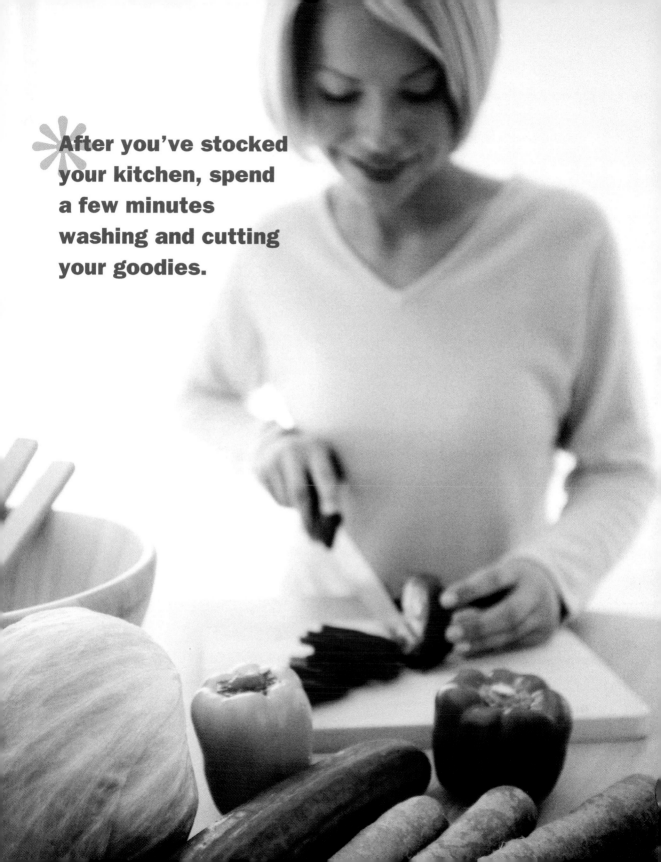

After you've stocked your kitchen, spend a few minutes washing and cutting your goodies.

Roasted Garlic Soup, which is lovely as a soup but delicious on anything as a sauce. You can season the dish yourself with fresh herbs and spices.

Cook up a batch of your own soups with low-sodium vegetable, chicken or beef stock as a base. You can also make your own stock or use the reserved liquid of cooked vegetables. Soups are a superb way of getting loads of vegetables into you.

Don't buy prepackaged, preseasoned grains. Always buy them plain so there are no extra hidden fats, sugars or salt.

Choose pastas made from grains rather than wheat or egg flour. There are delicious varieties made with spelt, kamut and rice. These are often easier to digest than wheat pastas and you can't taste the difference. Stick to vegetable-based pasta sauces. Add a lean grilled chicken breast for lean protein. A salad of mixed vegetables and greens makes a quick, healthy Clean-Eating meal.

PLANNED LEFTOVERS

One of my favorite ways to survive meal making is to prepare planned leftovers. My mom hated leftovers and always made someone in the family finish the last bits in the bowl rather than find a container and put it in the fridge. Not me! I love leftovers. I live on leftovers! I need leftovers!

So with a passion for leftovers I make them on purpose. Why make one chicken breast when you can make six? I grill several at a time and that way I

FLAVOR BOOSTERS NOT FAT BOOSTERS

Clean foods should be tasteful, not boring. Taste buds awaken to an intensified sense of food once you have started Eating Clean.

- Low-sodium bouillon cubes
- Low-sodium chicken, vegetable or beef broth
- Unsweetened applesauce
- Cranberry sauce
- Herbs, fresh and dried
- Horseradish
- Ketchup – look for brands with little or no added sugar
- Lemon juice
- Lime juice
- Garlic – fresh, frozen or dried
- Mustards
- Salsa
- Low-sodium soy sauce
- Spices
- Vinegars
- Worcestershire sauce
- Sea salt

have a number of meals ready to go. Roast a whole skinless turkey breast and slice it up. The slices make it easy to throw together a stir-fry in a pinch, or build a wrap for lunch or several lunches.

Toss whole grains, including rice, quinoa, barley or oatmeal in a slow cooker or rice steamer for plenty of accessible accompaniments to protein and complex carbohydrates. Buy enough ground turkey or chicken to make several patties or meatballs. These can be eaten warm for a delicious dinner with whole grains, yams or vegetables but are excellent cold and sliced into a wrap for lunch. Rely on nutritious homemade soups loaded with vegetables and whole grains for a quick lunch or a complete meal.

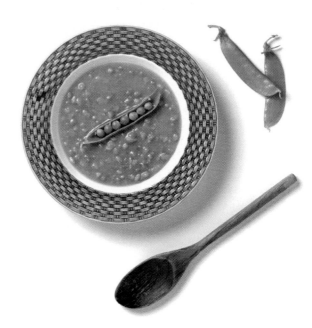

BUILDING A BETTER SANDWICH

Stop dreaming of an enormous club sandwich dripping with fatty ingredients and mayonnaise. There are numerous delicious ways to build a Clean-Eating sandwich. Keep your mind open to new ideas.

SWITCH IT	EAT IT
White bread	Whole or multi-grain high-fiber bread, pitas, wraps
Butter, mayo	Low-fat hummus, mustard, salsa, horseradish
Cheese	Low-fat cheese, goat cheese, low-fat cream cheese
Dressing	Moisten things up with salsa, sliced avocado, fresh tomato, lettuce, spinach leaves,cukes, grated carrot or sprouts, balsamic vinegar, mustard, lemon juice
Outside the box	Try whole-grain leftovers like rice, quinoa or couscous in a wrap

SEASONINGS & STAPLES

⋯⟩ **Fresh or dried herbs**

⋯⟩ **Sea salt** – it's the best and contains no added chemicals

⋯⟩ **Spices** – buy small amounts so you always have fresh on hand

⋯⟩ **Dried, frozen and fresh garlic**

⋯⟩ **Whole-wheat bran**

⋯⟩ **Oat bran**

⋯⟩ **Wheat germ**

⋯⟩ **Flaxseed**

⋯⟩ **Malt vinegar**

⋯⟩ **Rice vinegar**

⋯⟩ **Apple cider vinegar**

⋯⟩ **Balsamic vinegar, both white and dark**

⋯⟩ **Extra virgin olive oil**

⋯⟩ **Sesame oil**

⋯⟩ **Safflower oil**

⋯⟩ **Unsalted raw almonds, cashews, walnuts**

⋯⟩ **Raw unsalted sesame, pumpkin, and poppy seeds**

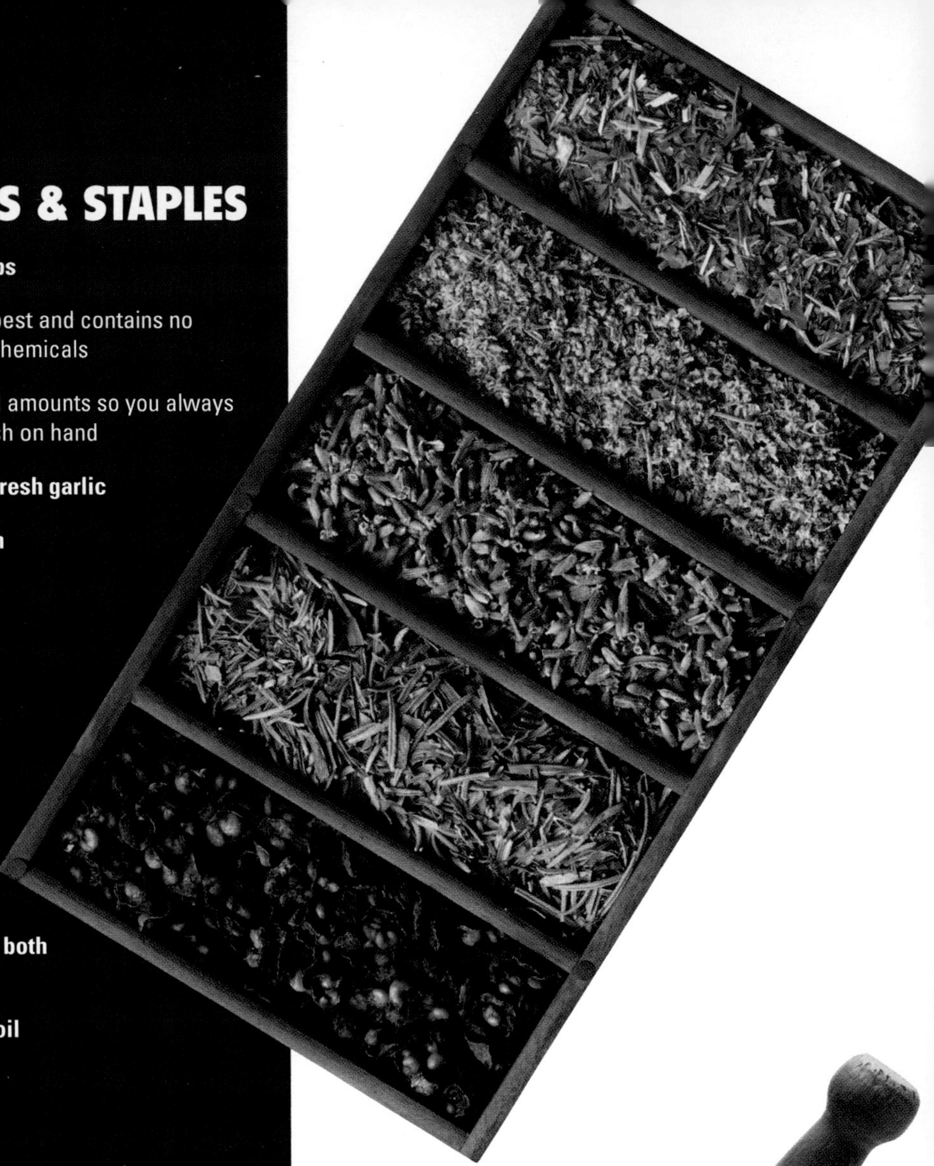

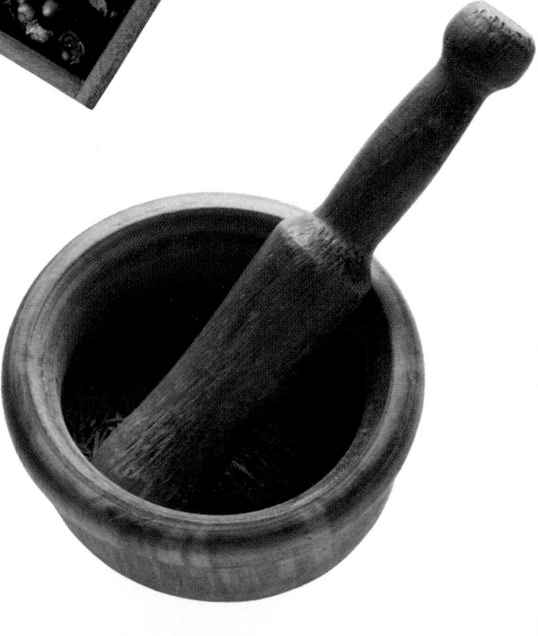

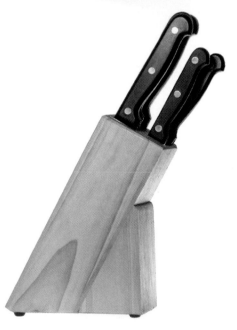

- **Good quality knives**

- **Food processor and/or a mini chopper**

- **Cutting boards** – nylon are best since they are more easily cleaned

- **Vegetable steamer**

- **Rice steamer**

- **Metal racks** – prevent meats from sitting in a pool of grease while cooking

- **Set of good-quality pans with tight-fitting lids**

- **Skillets in various sizes**

- **Roasting pans**

- **Casserole dishes with lids**

- **Nonstick bakeware**

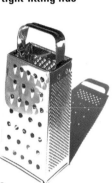

- **Mixing bowls**

- **Mixing cups and bowls**

- **Dry and liquid measuring cups**

- **Grater**

- **Wooden spoons for mixing**

- **Electric mixer**

- **Rubber spatulas**

- **Silpat sheets for nonstick baking**

- **Storage containers and food wrap**

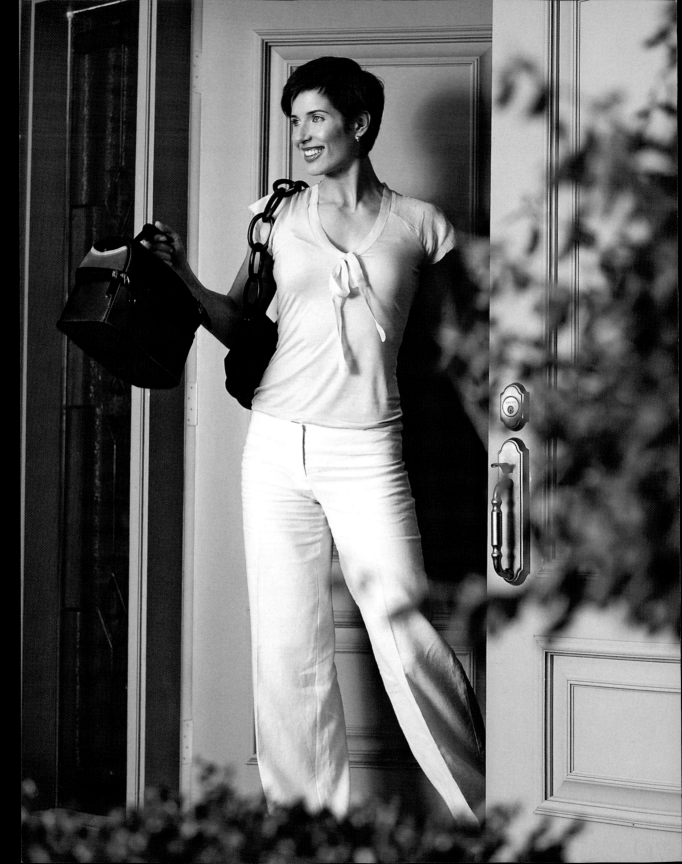

CHAPTER SIX

PACKING A
COOLER

CARRY IT!

In the early days on this continent First Nations peoples venturing on long hunting trips prepared foods to sustain them while they were gone. Riding on horseback across a vast plain they did not often come across McDonald's, open 24 hours per day, grilling hamburgers for takeout. No, First Nations peoples planned ahead so they wouldn't go hungry. Carrying food was simply a way of life, and one that made survival either possible or not.

If you're planning on going out for a day-long sail, the same applies. You must pack your food and provisions. There are no restaurants in the middle of open water! Do the same any time you jump in the car with family or friends for a hike, day trip, or even to work or school – you pack a cooler. It's the natural and smart thing to do. Many outdoor lovers know the value of having trail mix, water, energy bars and oranges tucked away in their backpack. These foods contribute to a more enjoyable experience. In my house if my family and I are not fed and watered regularly, we get cranky.

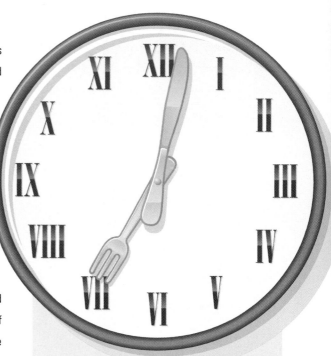

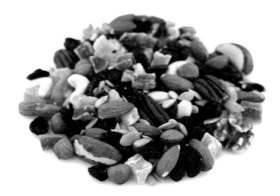

> **"One of the main rules of eating clean is that you must eat every two or three hours."**

COOLER PLANS EXPLAINED

The cooler plans below are meant for a day's worth of food. Choose the cooler that is right for you at this time. Read over the Eat-Clean Diet Principles on page 23 and refer to this checklist when packing your cooler:

⭐ Eat a combination of lean protein and complex carbohydrates at each meal.

⭐ Eat a meal every two – three hours.

⭐ Eat 5 – 6 meals each day.

⭐ Use portion sizes laid out on page 39.

⭐ If you are still genuinely hungry increase your portion sizes very slightly.

⭐ If you are not hungry within three hours then decrease your portion sizes slightly.

⭐ It's best if you can stop eating a few hours before bedtime, but if you are truly hungry (and not on the cooler-one plan) then you can eat a small meal before bed.

* If you are a vegetarian please refer to page 25 for lean protein options.

COOLER PLAN #1

HARDCORE EATING FOR RAPID RESULTS

WHAT IT'S FOR:

✔ Breaking plateaus
✔ The last 5 to 10 pounds
✔ Early contest preparation
✔ Photo shoots
✔ Showing increased muscular definition
✔ Quick weight loss

* Cooler one can be followed for a maximum of two weeks at a time.

* Eat your last meal at 6 pm, or four hours before bed.

WHAT IT IS:

Please note that this is the strictest of the cooler plans and will not be easy for some of you. There is very little room for indulgence and you may feel a little foggy due to lack of complex carbs. If it is too much you can add more complex carbohydrates (yam, apple, or brown rice) to one of your early meals. BUT hardcore eating promises results, and that is what you will get!

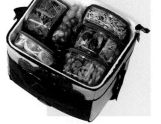

HOW IT WORKS:

(for a menu-plan example see page 182)

COMPLEX CARBOHYDRATES FROM FRUIT:

➜ 1 apple or pear per day (½ in the morning and ½ in the afternoon or evening).

COMPLEX CARBOHYDRATES FROM VEGETABLES (RAW OR STEAMED):

➜ 2 cupped handfuls eaten five times per day of cucumbers, radishes, tomatoes, leafy greens, broccoli, spinach, asparagus, green beans, sprouts, celery, bok choy, or other high-water content, non-starchy, low-glycemic index vegetables.

COMPLEX CARBOHYDRATES FROM WHOLE GRAINS AND STARCHY CARBOHYDRATES:

➜ 1 handful per day of cooked quinoa, brown rice, oatmeal, millet, or Cream of Wheat.
❖ Top this with:
  • 2 to 4 tablespoons of ground flaxseed
  • 2 to 4 tablespoons of bee pollen
➜ 1 hand-sized sweet potato or yam serving per day (½ in the morning and ½ in the afternoon or evening).

LEAN PROTEIN:

➜ 1 palm-sized portion eaten five or six times each day of chicken, tuna, egg whites, turkey, bison, elk, non-oily fish.
➜ Good-quality, sugar- and chemical-free protein powder (hemp, soy, or whey) may be substituted for any protein serving.

BEVERAGES:

➜ 1 gallon per day of distilled water, fresh water with no sodium, or clear, herbal tea (unsweetened).

AVOID:

✘ Dairy products
✘ Juice
✘ Bread
✘ Salad dressings – except lemon juice and balsamic vinegar
✘ Spreads (margarine, butter, mayonnaise, etc.)
✘ High-sodium foods

COOLER PLAN #2

WHAT IT'S FOR:

✔ Steady weight loss

✔ Maintenance once your goal weight is reached

WHAT IT IS:

This IS Eating Clean. Do this year round for steady, healthy weight loss. But this plan can also be used for maintenance. Here's why: when your body begins approaching its set point (its genetically predetermined healthy weight) you will find the weight loss will slow or stop.

The occasional treat (glass of wine, piece of chocolate, etc.) is permitted in limited amounts. Unhealthy sugars and fats are not recommended.

HOW IT WORKS:

(for a menu-plan example see page 184)

COMPLEX CARBOHYDRATES FROM FRUIT AND VEGETABLES: 6 portions each day. A portion is:

→ 1 cupped handful or piece of fruit, especially berries, grapefruit, melon, apples, mangoes.

→ 2 cupped handfuls of vegetables including broth-based / vegetable puree soups.

COMPLEX CARBOHYDRATES FROM WHOLE GRAINS AND STARCHY CARBOHYDRATES:

2 – 4 portions each day. A portion is:

→ 1 scant handful of high-protein, sugar-free cold cereals, such as muesli and granola

→ 1 handful of cooked cereal (see Cooler 1)

→ 1 piece of whole-grain bread or seven-inch wrap

→ 1 handful-sized serving of sweet potato, yam, banana, corn, carrots or squash (see examples of starchy complex carbs on page 66)

LEAN PROTEIN:

5 – 6 portions each day. A portion is:

→ 1 cup / 1 handful of dairy products (low-fat soy, almond, hemp, rice or lactose-free milk, cottage cheese, kefir, yogurt cheese, plain, fat-free, sugar-free yogurt)

→ 1 scant handful of raw, unsalted nuts

→ 2 tablespoons of all-natural nut butters

→ 1 palm-sized portion of animal meats (see Cooler 1)

→ Good-quality, sugar- and chemical-free protein powder (hemp, soy, or whey)

→ For vegetarian options please see page 25.

BEVERAGES:

→ 2 – 3 liters per day of fresh water with no sodium

→ Clear herbal tea (unsweetened)

→ Black coffee (in moderation)

→ Green / black tea

SWEETENERS: USE THESE IN MODERATION.
AVOID ARTIFICIAL SWEETENERS.

→ Honey

→ Agave nectar

→ Stevia

→ Sucanat

→ Rapadura sugar

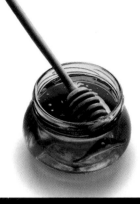

HEALTHY FATS: USE THESE IN MODERATION

→ Oils, especially olive, pumpkinseed, flaxseed, and safflower

→ Nuts and nut butters (see lean protein above)

→ Olive oil-based spreads

→ Fish and fish oils

Avoid:

✘ Juice

✘ Commercial salad dressings or sauces

✘ Fried, refined, and processed foods

COOLER PLAN #3

GETTING THE IDEA OF EATING FOR HEALTH AND LIFE

WHAT IT'S FOR:

✔ Getting used to the Clean-Eating lifestyle

WHAT IT IS:

This is Cooler #2 with more leniencies. If you are thinking about making changes to your current style of eating you may be wondering where to begin. Make some of these changes to your current food choices to introduce your body to Eating Clean.

For many of you, especially newcomers, Eating Clean will be a departure from any dieting or eating you have done before. You will need to make some changes right away so that you can begin to understand and experience the way Eating Clean can positively affect your health and body.

These are gentle changes, but still powerful enough that you will soon see results. What may be the big-

gest surprise is how good natural foods will taste once you begin to toss out the rest.

HOW IT WORKS:

Follow the Eat-Clean Principles on page 23.

EAT:

→ Oatmeal cooked with milk and sweetened with unsweetened applesauce or other fruits

→ High-protein, sugar-free cereals

→ Homemade soups and stews

→ Plenty of fresh fruits and vegetables

→ Low-fat cheese

→ Leaner cuts of meats with no obvious fat. Grill, broil or bake these options.

→ Beverages: clear, herbal teas, green/black tea, black coffee, 1 gallon of water (sodium free), fruit juice cut with water

AVOID:

- ✘ Unhealthy fats, especially butter, margarine, lard, cream, ice cream, fatty dressings, sauces, and meats
- ✘ Whole eggs (one may be eaten each day with egg whites)
- ✘ White table sugar
- ✘ Refined and processed foods
- ✘ Junk and fast foods
- ✘ Fried foods
- ✘ Excessive salt and sodium
- ✘ Excessive alcohol intake

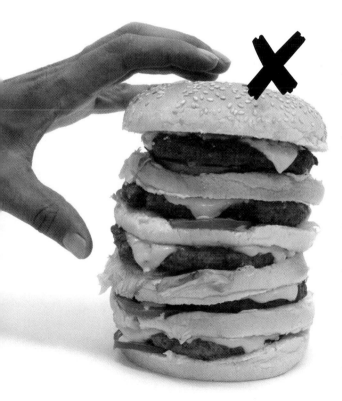

PACK A COOLER EVERY DAY

Success with Clean Eating demands that you pack a cooler every day. That makes sense when you think about one of the main rules of Eating Clean: you must eat every two to three hours. With that kind of eating frequency there's no question about it. Packing a cooler loaded with delicious, nutritious Clean-Eating foods is a safeguard against unhealthy food choices and cements your desire to make healthier eating decisions. That cooler will also keep you from overeating or munching on nutrient-poor treats.

I find having a cooler also prevents me from eating poorly when I am ravenous. It isn't fun to be hungry. You want something to eat and you want it fast. If your cooler is handy you will always have the luxury of Clean foods at your fingertips, and you'll have no reason to reach for that candy bar or bag of Doritos to fill the empty space.

HOW?

There are several ways to approach packing your cooler. The kinds of foods you pack determine how tight your nutrition will be, and also your desired rate of weight loss if that is part of your plan.

The first thing to remember is that all three coolers contain Clean Foods. Depending upon your goals you will choose one of the three plans to follow. The cooler plans are set up to give you a specific result. I have found this is necessary because some people need time to get into the habit of Clean Eating while others don't. Some want to lose fat, while others just want to get healthy. Cooler Plan Number One is very tight, and for most people not the easiest way to eat. You will likely be hungry. Cooler Plan Number Three is far less strict and helps to ease a newcomer to the realities of Clean Eating.

Creating three different plans allows you to choose how tight you want to keep your nutrition and the rate of weight loss you would like to experience. Clean Eating should help you lose a healthy amount of weight each week – an average of two to three pounds.

YOU WANT ME TO WHAT?

I know what you are thinking because I can almost hear the sighs and groans. "You want me to whaaat? Pack a cooler every day?" Yes that's right. Every day! Many of you will think it's too much work, and initially it may seem that way. But after you have adopted the habit into your lifestyle it becomes as easy as brushing your teeth. Besides, I've got loads of tips to help you learn how to do it and do it well. It's simple.

GETTING STARTED

Getting started with Clean-Eating cooler plans is fun. You are engaging in a new activity that holds a sense of promise, much like the sense of promise of reading a good book on summer vacation. You

need to start by making a few purchases. Visit your local big-box department store, hardware store or outdoor goods store. There you should find coolers of all sizes. Obviously you don't need a jumbo-sized version. Look for a soft-sided cooler measuring just large enough to handle three or four small meals. I like the ones with a hard plastic insert that slips out easily for washing. Most coolers of this size have an adjustable strap, making them easy to carry around.

While you're in the cooler section pick up a few ice packs. Re-freezable ones are best. I always buy a few extras because for some reason unknown to me they always go missing, just like socks in the drier. Having a few in your freezer is a good idea.

Once you've chosen these items you'll need an assortment of re-sealable containers in which to pack your meals. Here's a little tip I learned the hard way – choose containers with see-through lids and bottoms. It makes life much easier, especially when you're in a hurry in the morning, rushing around packing your cooler. Once I grabbed a container that I thought was filled with grilled chicken breasts only to find when I opened the container later in the day that it was full of uncooked pancake batter! Pretty disappointing when your stomach is growling like crazy and you come up empty. Containers with clear lids allow you to readily see what's inside.

Don't forget to pack a few incidentals such as napkins, travel wipes and cutlery. Now that you're set you can go home and get organized for the next big step – what to put in that cooler!

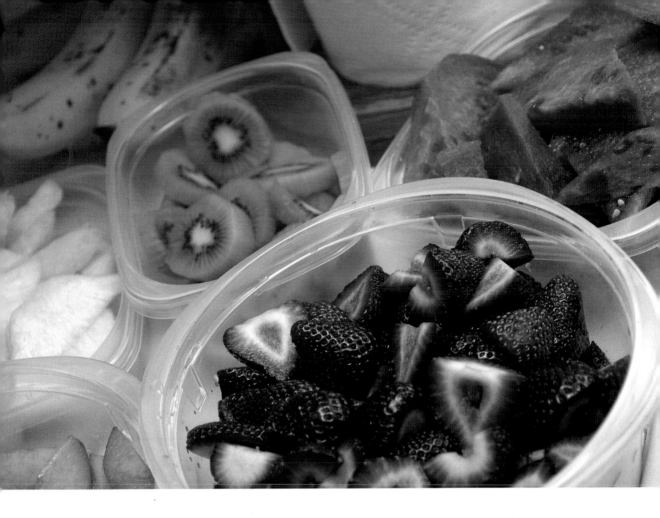

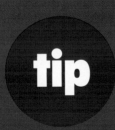 **tip**

Choose containers with see-through lids and bottoms.

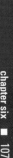

WHAT DO I PACK?

It is not difficult to pack a cooler when you have the right skills and a refrigerator full of good eats to help you sail through it. One of the most important tips you will learn is to make "Planned Leftovers." In other words, never grill just one chicken breast when you can grill several. That way you'll have enough for a few days and the planning of mealtimes becomes a much simpler task.

Similarly, you can roast a few pork tenderloins or one whole lean turkey breast, even a few salmon steaks. That way you will always have sufficient lean protein to choose from when planning meals for a day. Here's another trick: don't just boil one egg; boil the whole dozen. Boiled eggs keep well for a few days and are a simple, reliable complete protein source. Water-packed tuna is a cinch, especially now that you can purchase it in small pouches that don't require a can opener. Very portable! Stock your cupboards with loads of salmon too.

Made a stew last night? Pack a serving of that. Anything you can eat, you can pack. And make sure to pack your complex carbs. Brown rice, sweet potato, whole-grain breads and wraps are all good starchy carb choices, and a great big salad along with a couple of pieces of fruit round out the day.

While you pack your cooler, make sure to pair your complex carbs with your lean protein so you know you have what you need for each meal.

EATING CLEAN— SIMPLE, NOT BORING, EAT MORE FOOD, NOT LESS

It's easy to think Clean Eating is a boring way to eat because the varieties of foods seem limited. In fact, just the opposite is true. Clean, wholesome foods can be prepared and served in countless delicious ways. Nutrition based on Clean-Eating principles is exciting and always interesting. How can wholesome fruits and vegetables ever be boring? Just holding a crisp red apple or a juicy mango in your hand makes you feel healthier. Compare that to the way you feel as you unwrap a grease-soaked hamburger and bite into its soggy white bun. The food sits like lead in

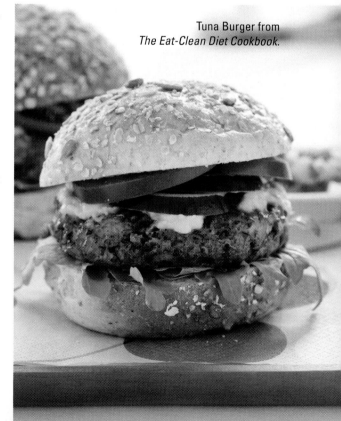

Tuna Burger from
The Eat-Clean Diet Cookbook.

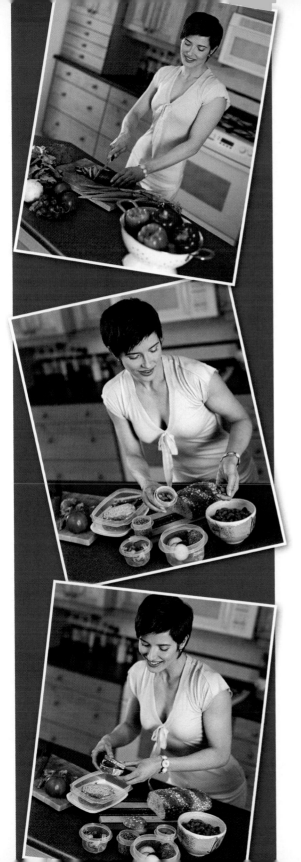

your stomach — not appetizing at all. Try a salmon or chicken breast burger instead. Make your beef lean and omit greasy fast-food options. The Tuna Burger in my Eat-Clean Diet Cookbook is delish!

EATING CLEAN — A CINCH

I think of Eating Clean as a relief. Why? Following the Clean-Eating plan is like following a map. I know what food choices to make, how much to eat and when to eat it, so I never guess about meals. By combining complex carbohydrates from fruits, vegetables and whole grains with lean protein, every meal is laid out before me. I find the more structure I have around meals and meal preparation the more likely I am to stick with this kind of lifestyle eating.

SUCCESS IS PREPARATION

Eating Clean is much easier if you are prepared. You need to have a good supply of Clean-Eating foods in your fridge and cupboard and packed in your cooler to really make it work! Doing a little pre-shopping planning helps you get what need when you finally arrive at the supermarket. I like to look at various magazines for recipe ideas. I also check out the local farmers' markets and go crazy with local produce, particularly that which is in season. Foods in season always taste better, ensuring mealtime success.

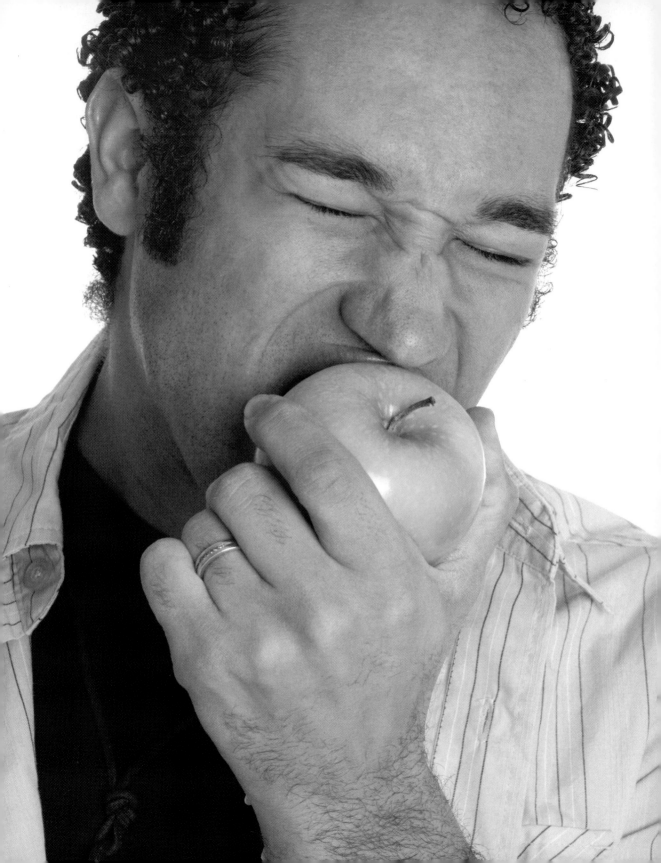

CHAPTER SEVEN

MEN CAN EAT CLEAN TOO

Okay guys, it's your turn. I have received this question from men too many times: "Is Clean Eating for me?" Relax! Men can jump on Clean Eating because doing so does not mean dieting. Most "diets" are far too restrictive and low in calories for men to follow, but following these principles of eating can be thought of as a lifestyle. This is something you live with, not a temporary fix. Servings are based on body size, not on some arbitrary number. You hear your wives or girlfriends talking diet all the time. Who needs more of that? So Clean Eating it is!

You will be in good company, since many men are already enjoying the Clean-Eating lifestyle. This new way of eating originated in the sport of men's bodybuilding, where men sought to define muscle by chasing fat from their body. Muscle doesn't show appreciably unless bodyfat levels are in the single digits, so competitive bodybuilders had to develop the best and most reliable method for losing bodyfat. And they had to do this while retaining their muscle mass and energy, whereas most diets deplete both. Of course in the bodybuilding world this eating regimen is taken to the extreme. You will likely choose not to keep your nutrition as tightly in check as a competitive bodybuilder does, but you should find it encouraging to learn that these gentle giants are eating the same way you are. You will be in good company.

MEN ARE DIFFERENT

I have to start with a generalization although it is terribly cliché but I'll take the risk. I am sure there are

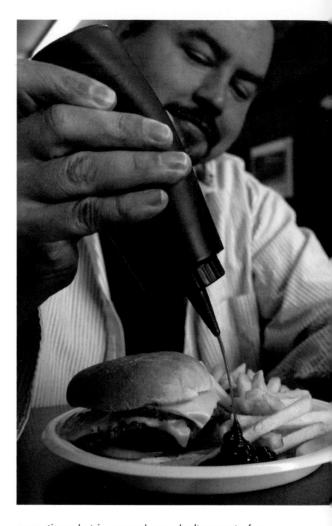

exceptions, but in general men don't seem to fuss over details about nutrition as much as women do. Foodies may disagree, but I feel my thinking is sound as I have witnessed this myself. The way men are wired seems to make them more concerned about how the car is functioning than how their own body is functioning. In part this is because most men have their meals prepared by a wife, partner or mother. Food is a consideration only when a man is hungry and often anything will do as long as it is food. Witness the ultimate man's meal-in-a-hurry: a plate of nachos, chased with a beer.

What questions would a man have to ask himself if his food was served to him daily, whether by a wife, mother, or waitress? Not many. Someone prepares the food in question puts it on a plate and sets it in front of said man. The food is consumed, the meal is over and that is the end of it. This goes on ad infinitum or until there is some sort of crisis – preferably a clothing malfunction, as in when favorite pants no longer zip up, but possibly a grave health crisis.

THEY LOVE IT!

I do realize there are many men who defy this generalization – my brothers and my husband for example. They not only take a keen interest in food, new ingredients and their health, but they even like cooking. One brother, Rene, created an apricot chicken recipe that he served to many young women when he was at the dating stage of his life. Now he is as likely as his beautiful wife Jody to prepare dinner for his family. When summer is over and there is a bounty of vegetables in his garden, Rene cooks up an enormous batch of tomato sauce and preserves it for use during the winter. Ron, our elder brother, has a vegetable garden as well, and he is in charge of what goes in and what comes out of it. He loves to grill and enjoys eating nutritious, high-quality foods with his family too. His wife Tammy, a distance athlete, depends on excellent nutrition for conditioning.

My brothers may be exceptions to the rule but I do know they share a love of cooking and clean food. And of course my husband Eats Clean as if it's his religion, to keep lean and strong.

EAT MORE

One of the main principles of Eating Clean is that you eat more. I don't know too many diets that tell you to do this! When Eating Clean you eat every three hours. That means you never go hungry. Many diets depend on deprivation, reducing food intake and, even worse, counting calories. Most men I know don't like to go hungry – they love to eat! And they HATE counting calories. Clean Eating does not involve any of this nonsense. It is simply a way of eating

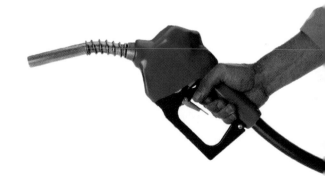

that embraces the healthiest of foods, which are eaten steadily throughout the day to refuel the body. Aren't you relieved?

I like to say you can compare Clean Eating to fueling a high-performance sports car. Imagine a sleek new Jaguar XJ. When it's time to gas up you don't pump regular gas into the tank. Now think of your body as a high-performance vehicle. You don't want to pump it full of low-grade fuel do you? When you consume a steady diet of simple carbohydrates (sugars), greasy fats and processed foods you are filling your (irreplaceable) high-performance vehicle, aka your body, with garbage-quality, lowest-grade fuel. You can't expect to perform well when you ask your body to operate on junk. Slowly it will begin to deteriorate, become sluggish and eventually falter.

The foods recommended for Clean Eating are nutrient dense. You can consider them your high-octane body fuel. The foundation of this lifestyle way of eating is a platform of protein. Protein is the single most important macronutrient for building and maintaining a healthy, strong physique. However, protein must always be partnered with complex carbohydrates for optimum physical performance. Together they

Protein must always be partnered with complex carbohydrates for optimum physical performance.

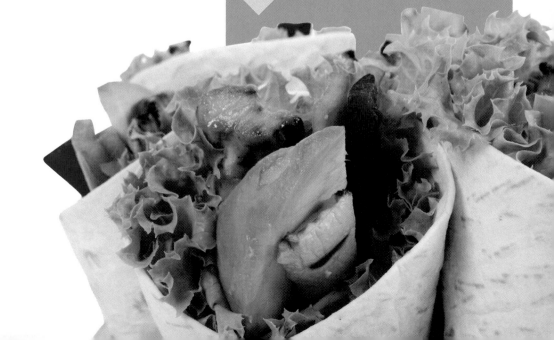

burn slowly and efficiently as they are processed. Your lunch, for example, might include a grilled skinless chicken breast tucked into a multigrain wrap that has been spread with hummus and is further stuffed with baby spinach, sprouts and sliced tomato. Delicious! Food like this means you will always have a steady supply of energy to get through your day. Food like this also mean you won't be heavy and sluggish. And food like this tastes incredible.

WHAT'S LUNCH GOT TO DO WITH IT?

Contrast a delicious lunch like that with normal lunchtime fare – fries and a burger with a jumbo soda. If you happen to be dining on the newest Monster Thickburger from Hardee's – an SUV-sized hunk of meat and dressings – you will be gorging on 1410 calories, 107 grams of fat, 45 grams of saturated fat and 2740 milligrams of sodium. That's before adding the fries and soda. And that's not even the worst version of this backyard favorite. The Double Six Dollar burger from Carl's Jr. contains 1520 calories, 111 grams of fat, 47 grams of saturated fat and 2760 milligrams of sodium. These sandwiches are heart attacks on a plate, and definitely not Clean-Eating foods.

CARRY IT!

Another critical Clean-Eating principle is to eat regularly. Eating several small meals per day will necessitate carrying lunch and other small meals with you to work. Most men don't like carrying lunch pails. But my dad went to work every day with a lunch pail. Yours probably did too. A Thermos full of hot tea and many other delicious eats went into his lunch pail to sustain him through his busy day. Back then all men carried their lunch with them. My brother-in-law, Warren, carries a similar lunch pail and Thermos on his job. My brothers opt for brown-bag lunches, which they pack themselves in the morning. These days there are plenty of cooler options available to carry your lunch in. In fact, you may have used one of these coolers to carry a six-pack to the park or beach.

However you choose to carry your food you will have to do so in order to keep yourself on track with Clean Eating. Bringing lunch ensures that you will have a supply of healthy food options handy just when the hunger pangs start up. If you don't the chance is far greater that you will stand in line at a fast-food place ordering up mega BAD sandwiches.

CLEAN EATING, SO WHAT?

A steady diet of low-grade fuels saturated with unhealthy fats, processed and chemically charged ingredients and too much sugar coupled with a lack of exercise makes for trouble. This trouble can present itself in many serious ways including diabetes, pre-diabetes, metabolic syndrome X, heart attack, stroke, hypertension, arthritis, breathing disorders and cancer. Excess weight and poor nutrition affect the body in so many detrimental ways, the list can go on indefinitely.

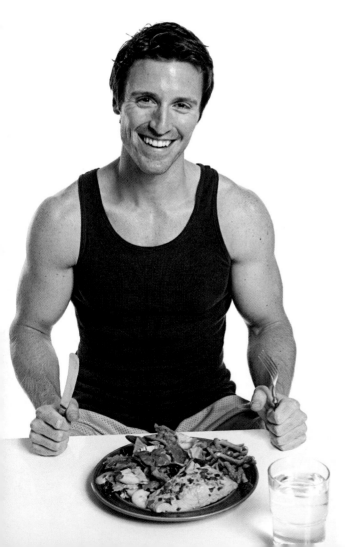

> **"Good nutrition will also help you immensely when combating diseases that are genetically programmed to occur."**

Health shouldn't be taken for granted. Life is a joyous experience. To be given the gift of a brand new day every morning, to know you are able bodied and minded and to know the joy of love and being loved are exactly the right reasons to look after yourself in the best possible way with Clean Eating. If you have spent any time in a hospital even just as a visitor you will need no further reminding of how horrible life can be if you don't take care. I doubt anyone can say they have had a pleasant stay while parked in a hospital room.

Clean Eating is your daily prevention against such possibilities. It won't prevent every kind of illness because some are genetically programmed, but giving your body Clean-Eating perfect nutrition is the only way to eat and the best way to prevent trouble as much as you possibly can. Good nutrition will also help you immensely when combating diseases that are genetically programmed to occur. If you keep up with fast-food feedings, you will inevitably end up overweight and sick.

MIKEY LIKES IT!

As with any new way of eating, the big question is: "If it's healthy will it taste good?" Many of you think that eating healthy means it has to taste like cardboard. I don't much like the taste of cardboard, so I don't blame you on that count. But you can rest easy. Clean Eating tastes far superior to any other way of eating. That's because the food you are eating is not jacked up with chemicals and garbage. How can you improve on the flavor of a fresh tomato, plump and juicy from the vine or ripened on your windowsill? The entire scope of the produce section is available to you for your selection of complex carbohydrates from fruit and vegetables. You also have a huge array of other complex carbs to choose from, such as brown rice, sweet potatoes and other grains and starchy vegetables. Partner those with lean protein from meats, fish, dairy and non-meat sources and you have the beginnings of a seriously delicious meal. Now up the ante with spices, herbs, citrus fruits, vinegars and oils and you are really turning up the heat on flavor.

HOW WILL YOU FEEL?

Initially if you have been depending on a family-sized bag of Doritos for your weekend nutrition you may have a few rough spots ahead. The body will go through a detox. The symptoms of your detox will vary, depending on how heavy your snack and bad-food habit has been. You may feel a little shaky, headachy and not quite yourself, but none of this is serious. You will get through it and once you have come through the detox and out the other side you will be the better for it. In fact, you will likely be amazed at how much energy you have. Hang tough! You can do it!

Many of you will have no discomfort at all. You will simply change your food choices, eat more and eat more regularly. The great majority of you will find yourselves feeling much better. With continued Clean Eating you will have increased energy and experience more regular bowel function. You will also find that your blood pressure will improve, dropping back into the healthy range. You may be able to reduce your intake of blood-pressure medication. Many men have found that with Clean Eating they can control their symptoms of diabetes, and often reduce or even omit insulin altogether. The same is true of heart medication. Naturally any changes in medication will have to be done under your doctor's supervision and with his advice.

As a bonus: if all these systems are working properly thanks to improved nutrition, there is a very good chance your sexual health will also improve. Much of the workings of the sex organs have to do with blood pressure and cardio function.

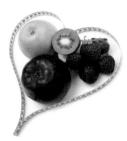

CLEAN EATING IS FOR MEN

Now you know. Clean Eating is absolutely for men. The principles are not difficult to incorporate into your lifestyle, and soon enough they will become your lifestyle. When eating turns into a healthy way of life you will be set up for long-term success. Your struggles with what to eat, how to eat and when to eat will be over and so will your battle with weight. Clean Eating is the only way to eat.

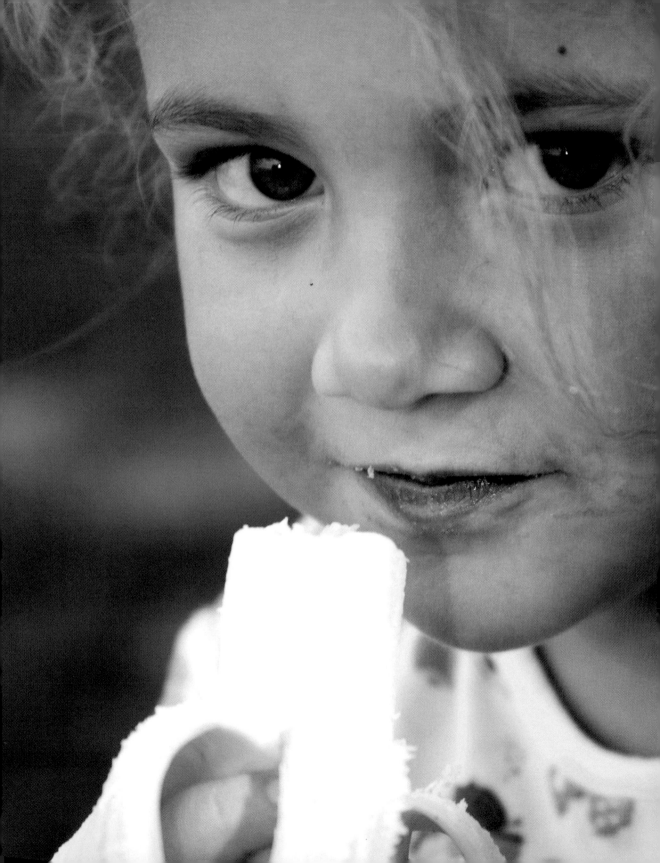

CHAPTER EIGHT

EAT-CLEAN
KIDS

When I began my journey with Clean Eating I met with resistance from my family. My three daughters, extremely active in competitive dance and school sports, were not overweight and never thought twice about what they put in their mouth. They were used to me being the Martha Stewart-type mom who did a lot of home baking, home-cooked meals and other activities centered around food.

Family gatherings of 24 or more were common at our home. Often the celebration, whether it was a birthday, major holiday or other festivity, focused on the "potluck, what can you bring?" style of eating. That meant the meal could run the gamut of offerings, from mayonnaise-laden salads to potatoes loaded with sour cream to deep-fried chicken wings to buttery, sugary desserts. At these gatherings, the healthiest Clean-Eating food you could hope for would be a platter of raw veggies and dip. No one really thought much about Clean Eating.

HEALTHY FOOD ISN'T HEALTHY

In fact, at our gatherings people often claimed they were eating healthy. While they were telling you this they would be munching on a pasty white bun loaded with margarine or butter, cheese and deli meats. Yes, it sounds healthy but on closer inspection that "healthy" sandwich proves to be groaning with unnecessary saturated fats, sugars and calories. I mean, it's obvious when you're eating a half bag of Doritos you're eating junk and you know you're doing it because, well, it's junk food. But the deli sandwich contains as much unhealthy fat and sugar as the junk food. Toss in a Coke and you've made things worse. Sometimes we are misled by the notion we are eating healthily when we're not. Potluck suppers like the ones I often hosted were a minefield of unhealthy eating choices.

Proper nutrition is the largest component of shaping a better physique.

HOW DO YOU GET YOUR KIDS TO COME ALONG FOR THE RIDE?

If you have children it makes sense to teach them how to Eat Clean right along with you. If they are young Eating Clean will be the only way they know how to eat. You will be setting the example for them after reading this book. Older children will come to appreciate the benefits of healthier eating, including clean and glowing skin, beautiful shiny hair, improved energy and super-charged brain function. Most kids eat whatever is presented to them – that goes for good food or garbage – because they trust Mom and Dad to put good food on the table. It's the job of parents (mostly) to offer and prepare foods that are nutritious and children assume that's what is happening.

WHAT ARE YOU USED TO?

If you have grown up exposed to sugary, greasy, over-processed refined foods – Froot Loops, donuts, danishes, chocolate milk, soda, fries, hamburgers, hotdogs and the like, you will think this is nutrition. You couldn't be blamed, either, because it is stuff you have considered to be food for as long as you know. Until this day! Now you are reading this book and you will come to understand that the only people who benefit from such nutrient-deficient foods are the big companies driven by the "Suits" who manufacture them.

Think about it; do Marshmallow Peeps fit anywhere in the food pyramid? What about Krispy Kreme donuts?

NUTRIENT-DENSE FOODS

With a little guidance you will soon see that Clean Eating promises to nourish the body with high-quality foods that feed every cell in every square inch of you. Nutrient-dense foods replenish the body and provide energy for maintenance, repair and growth and keep your body trim, well defined and strong. Proper nutrition is the largest component of shaping a better physique. Let me put that another way: Eat Clean. You'll feel great and look great too!

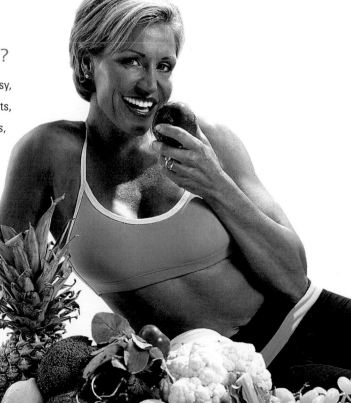

CLEAN EATING FOR YOU AND YOUR CHILDREN

Lately I have been invited to schools to give Clean-Eating seminars. Each time I have it has been a joyful experience for me. Students and teachers were keen to learn more about nutrition, which surprised me. I would look around the classroom or auditorium where I was presenting and see a crowd of kids leaning forward eagerly, wanting to learn as much as possible. I wasn't prepared for that. I thought I would be perceived as just another boring adult. Their enthusiasm energized me, helping me believe there really is a need to re-educate our youth and ourselves. Teachers smiled in the background approvingly. The teachers' job is made much easier when children come to school well nourished. And more students than you would imagine come to school with empty stomachs!

WHAT DID YOU HAVE FOR BREAKFAST?

I always start my seminar with a discussion about breakfast. "How many of you had breakfast before coming to school today?" I ask. Timid hands rise, and it doesn't take long before it is clear that sometimes only half the kids have managed to eat breakfast. The next question is always "Did anyone have hot cereal like oatmeal for breakfast?" I remember one kid saying he thought oats were for horses. Wasn't real cereal the kind you got out of a pretty colored box like Froot Loops? Most children identify breakfast with some sort of food that comes prepackaged with fun pictures on a box. Often these are sugar-loaded cereals, gooey pastries or greasy sausage creations. It's the rare kid who eats oatmeal. One little girl said she ate a double chocolate donut for breakfast every day, washed down with Pepsi.

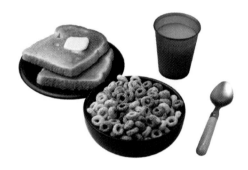

Most children identify breakfast with some sort of food that comes prepackaged with fun pictures on a box.

WE NEED TO KNOW

You see what I mean? There is a definite need to re-educate our children and ourselves about nutrition. The entire cold cereal aisle is set up to win kids over. Choosing cereal has nothing to do with Mom today. In our mother's times and those before her, Mom chose what the family ate. Now kids tell the mothers what to buy. They've seen the television commercials.

At this time in my presentation I dig into a bag packed with Clean-Eating foods. Pulling out apples I toss them into the audience. "Apples are the perfect snack food! They come in a neat package that makes an apple easily transportable. Apples are chock full of nutrition and they taste delicious." Kids love catching the apples and crunching into them while I talk. Then I launch into a discussion about junk foods prepared in disgusting saturated and trans fats, both of which cause damage to blood vessels and tissues. The students usually moan and groan out loud when I tell them this part.

START WITH BREAKFAST

Digging deeper into my tote I pull out a bag of oatmeal – not the instant kind. Along with it I pull out flaxseed, wheat germ and bee pollen. There is no better way to start the day than with these superior foods. Oatmeal is a breakfast superfood. Grandma knew what many before her knew, that whole-grain oatmeal was nutritious and kept the tummy full for long periods of time. So nourishing is the humble grain, it is one of the few whole foods recognized by the Food and Drug Administration as having medical benefits. It sports a health claim on its label as follows: "Diets low in saturated fat and cholesterol that include soluble fiber from oatmeal may reduce the risk of heart disease."

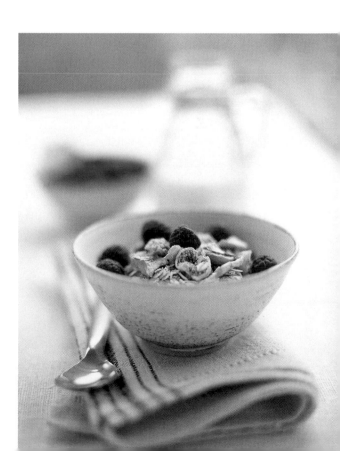

Today researchers have lots of scientific language explaining why the full feeling lasts longer from oatmeal and why the food is so good for you. One reason is that oatmeal is loaded with soluble fiber.

The soluble fiber even has a name – beta glucan. This stays in the tummy longer, prolonging the full feeling. That's good news for kids, especially those who are active. Your brain likes oatmeal too!

Another excellent argument for starting your day with a bowl of steaming oatmeal is that fiber helps control weight loss. And most of us don't consume enough fiber – the recommended daily amount is 25 to 35 grams. Recently the Food and Nutrition Board of the Institute of Medicine reported their recommended daily fiber intakes. For women aged 19 to 50 years of age, 25 grams per day is best. Women older than that should consume 21 grams. Men aged 19 to 50 years need 38 grams while older men do best with 30 grams.

Ref: Steven Pratt M .D. and Kathy Matthews, *SuperFoods – The Fourteen that will Change Your Life*, Harper, 2005

DON'T BE AFRAID

It is easy to talk to kids and introduce them to what amounts to a whole new way of eating in many cases. Kids are smart. Sometimes their parents either don't have time or simply don't know better. They see food at the grocery stores and put it on the table. Give your kids a chance and I think you'll find they are eager to eat healthy and clean just like you.

With three daughters I have plenty of traffic roaring through my house and subsequently many mouths to feed. The only kind of food I will prepare is clean food. That's what's served around here. Not only do my children now prefer it, their friends do too.

"Give your kids a chance and I think you'll find they are eager to eat healthy and clean just like you."

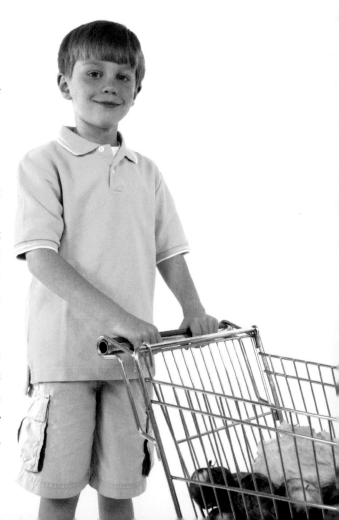

They will often go back to their parents saying they want to eat oatmeal for breakfast from now on. It's positive and encouraging to see kids so open minded but what I think they really like is the quality they get with Clean Eating. It just tastes so much better!

There is no need to be afraid of teaching your children how to Eat Clean. You aren't depriving them of valuable nutrients with this way of eating; you'll be giving them far more. Your children will have eating tools that will stand them in good stead for life. And remember Clean Eating is not just a traditional diet, it's a lifestyle. Wouldn't it be nice to know that the habits you are giving your kids will ensure that they never encounter the weight problems you have experienced?

HEALTHY HABITS

What's the best aspect of Clean Eating? The fact that it becomes a healthy habit is exceedingly valuable today in an age when our youth are succumbing to eating disorders at younger and younger ages and at alarming rates. All eating disorders stem from abnormal relationships with food. Several million North Americans suffer from some form of eating disorder. According to the National Association of Anorexia Nervosa and Associated Disorders, more than 1 in 10 high school students have an eating disorder. Millions more have binge-eating disorders. Millions again struggle with weight, body image and the consequences of these. Eating disorders, it seems, are never far away from your door.

Most eating disorders are efforts to control weight and environment, resulting in severely wasted physiques. The slang term "ANA," used by young girls today, is short for anorexia nervosa. It scares me to hear this term thrown around so casually. It sounds so innocent it seems like there's nothing wrong with deliberately starving oneself of food. In fact the consequences are dire and life threatening.

fact For the first time in history children may not live the long, healthy lives their parents did, thanks to poor nutritional habits.

WILL OUR CHILDREN SURVIVE?

On the other hand there are millions of North American youth and more worldwide who are overweight. Here's a sobering fact: for the first time in history children may not survive their parents because of overeating disorders. It has recently been suggested that at the same time baby boomers are experiencing their first heart attack around the age of 64, their children will be having their first heart attacks too. Heart attack is directly related to overweight and overweight comes from ... you guessed it, garbage food.

UNHEALTHY EATING HABITS

THE DISORDERS

- **Restriction:** severe limitation of food intake, starving, skipping or avoiding meals, regular use of appetite suppressants or fat burners to lose weight.

- **Overeating:** eating more than the body needs to sustain itself.

- **Purging:** use of over-the-counter drugs, laxatives (diarrhea), emetics (vomiting), diuretics (loss of fluids) to "rid" the body of food.

- **Excessive exercise.**

- **Spit chewed food out before swallowing.**

- **Deliberate dehydration.**

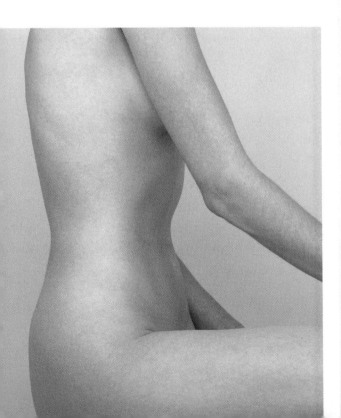

HERE ARE SOME TIPS ON HOW TO CREATE A HEALTHIER ATTITUDE TOWARDS FOOD IN YOUR CHILDREN

- **Set structured meal times.** If you set firm meal and snack times, then the goal is to stay with these times, within reason, over the long term.

- **Tell your children their bodies are terrific and healthy.** That doesn't mean you have to lie. Find their best features and flatter them. Teach them to be strong within themselves.

- **Teach your children that young bodies are constantly growing and developing and that change is normal.** Stress that all bodies are different and there is beauty in each difference.

- **Use scales once a week at the most.** Weighing yourself every day isn't necessary.

- **Offer varied choices of clean foods.** Allow your children to decide what they want to eat but make the offerings healthy and nutritious. Eliminate junk right at the grocery store.

- **Choose your battles.** Say yes occasionally to unhealthy treats. A treat means an indulgence eaten once in a while, not every day.

- **Bring both healthy snacks into your home and occasionally unhealthy ones.** Chances are they will prefer the healthier snacks.

- **Place a heavy emphasis on physical activity, including unstructured play.**

- **Take your children grocery shopping.**

- **Set the example yourself, every day.**

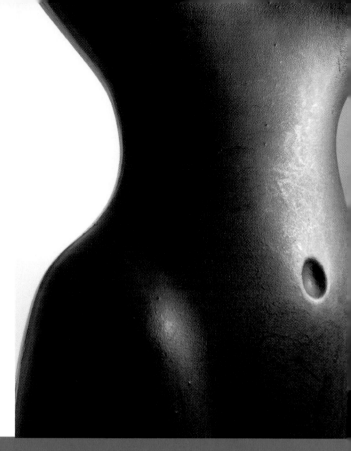

UNREALISTIC EXPECTATIONS

Magazine pictures are electronically edited and airbrushed yet teenagers (and adults) strive to look like these so-called perfect cover girls. Many entertainment celebrities are severely underweight. Some not only *look like* they have anorexia, they *do* have it. How do we really know what we should look like? It's confusing. The table below compares average women in the US with Barbie Doll and department store mannequins. It's not encouraging.

Ref: *Health Magazine*, September 1997; and NEDIC, a Canadian eating disorders advocacy group.

Many entertainment celebrities are severely underweight.

	AVERAGE WOMEN	BARBIE	STORE MANNEQUIN
HEIGHT	5'4"	6'0"	6'0"
WEIGHT	145lbs	101lbs	N/A
DRESS SIZE	12-14	4	6
BUST	36-37"	39"	34"
WAIST	29-31"	19"	23"
HIPS	40-42"	33"	34"

EAT AGAIN

I'll never forget one of the most meaningful experiences I had as a result of my passion for training and Clean Eating. An 18-year-old girl approached me, saying she wanted to thank me for my words. She had been reading my column, "Raise The Bar" in *Oxygen* magazine, especially while she was in the hospital. Apparently she had been hospitalized while recovering from anorexia. She had made sufficient strides after nearly losing her life but her words will stay with me forever. She said, *"Thank you for teaching me that it's okay to eat. Thank you for teaching me what a normal body image is. Thank you for telling me eating is better."* As she spoke her parents stood by weeping. This was their little girl who they nearly lost and who was still painfully thin but she was getting better because she was beginning to understand how to nourish herself properly. They were overjoyed. After the family left, I too cried.

EATING CLEAN— A HEALTHY HABIT

I am convinced Clean Eating is the answer to many eating disorders because it is a lifestyle and a set of easily practiced habits. And that's what eating should be, a healthy habit to sustain a normal, healthy body. In my opinion Clean Eating is a relief. It spells out clearly what is nutritious and what is not. It is based on whole foods with minimal goop to dress it up. It delivers all the essential macro and micro nutrients. It maintains steady levels of insulin so blood glucose levels do not swing wildly. Your metabolism stays charged by your eating every two to three hours. It keeps you well hydrated. Best of all, it is not a fad diet. There's no need to purchase fancy pre-packaged meals and tablets or go to meetings. It's a plan kids can easily follow with plenty of delicious foods to keep them healthy and happy.

HEALTH CONSEQUENCES FROM OVERWEIGHT OR OBESITY

- Risk of heart disease precursors including increased cholesterol and high blood pressure.
- Increase of type 2 diabetes
- Overweight kid = overweight adult
- Social discrimination

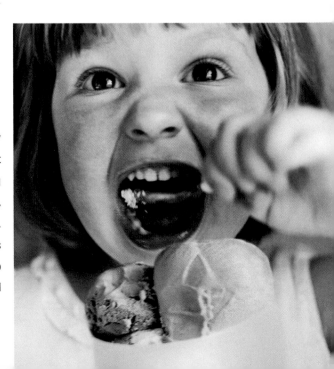

WE DON'T WANT JUNK!

Once your children start Eating Clean they will not enjoy junk food in the same way. That's a promise! Teenagers have notoriously poor eating habits. They feed voraciously on greasy French fries and sugar-loaded carbonated beverages and all manner of garbage foods. These foods will lose their appeal after Clean Eating has been implemented in your household. They won't taste good and in some cases they can make your child feel nauseated.

We have practised Clean Eating for six years now. It's extremely rare that my daughters go to McDonald's anymore, but if they do happen to go there the food always gives them a stomachache afterwards. Their tummies have not been exposed to the additives and grease, and so much garbage upsets their systems. They prefer to Eat Clean and always take their food with them in a cooler so they won't go hungry or be tempted to eat junk on the run.

GLOBESITY

More children than ever are overweight and even obese, with numbers reaching epidemic proportions. Increasing rates of overweight and obesity pave the way for increasing numbers of fat-related disease. Globally 22 million of the world's children under five years of age are overweight or obese. In North America 33 percent of children are overweight. Add to this the number of fat-related illnesses becoming more prevalent and it's clear our kids face enormous

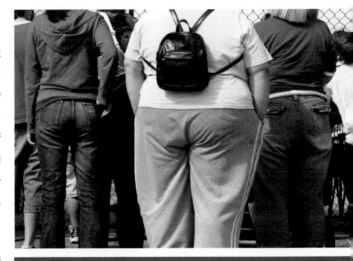

Globally **22 million** of the world's **children under five years of age are overweight or obese.**

health risks. Poor nutritional habits are clear cutting a path to illnesses including cancer, heart disease, diabetes and hypertension.

There is a strong argument here to introduce your child to Clean Eating. By doing so, you as a parent prevent many medical problems related to poor nutrition and eating disorders. The very thing that makes these kids so afraid of food is in fact the one thing that can save them and build a healthy, strong, ideal body, because Clean Eating does not involve avoiding any of the five macronutrients and six major food groups. Read that again. *Clean Eating does not advocate avoiding any of the six food groups, all of which are necessary for good health.*

THE SIX FOOD GROUPS

Oils

Whole Grains

Dairy

Vegetables

Fruits

Meat & Beans

www.mypyramid.gov

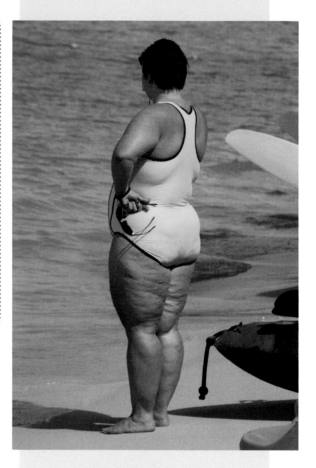

ADULT HEALTH CONSEQUENCES OF OVERWEIGHT

- Premature death.

- Even a modest 10 to 12 pounds of excess fat increases the risk of death, heart disease, high blood pressure and elevates triglycerides.

- Diabetes: a weight gain of 11 to 18 pounds increases risk of development of type 2 diabetes to double that of those who have not gained weight.

- 80 percent of people who are overweight have diabetes.

- Cancer: increased risk of endometrial, colon, gall bladder, prostate, kidney and post-menopausal cancer.

- Breathing problems like sleep apnea, asthma.

80%
of people who are **overweight** have **diabetes**

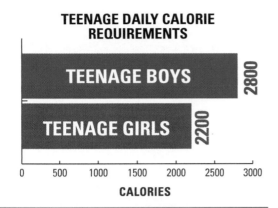

TEENAGE DAILY CALORIE REQUIREMENTS

TEENAGE BOYS — 2800

TEENAGE GIRLS — 2200

CALORIES

STATS

- More than 50 percent of teenaged girls think they should be on diets.

- 1 percent of female adolescents have anorexia– or 1 in every 100 young women between the ages of 10 to 20 are starving themselves.

- 4 out of 100 college-aged women have bulimia.

- 31 percent of North American teenage girls and 18 percent of boys are somewhat overweight.

- Another 15 percent of North American teenage girls and 14 percent of boys are obese.

CAUSES

- Excessive and ready access to junk food.

- Fewer home-cooked meals.

- More eating out.

- Too much snacking.

- Snack foods high in sugar and fat.

- Little or no physical activity.

- More driving, less walking.

- Increased time spent in front of the TV, computer or game console.

- More sedentary lifestyle.

SET THE EXAMPLE

Parents, the sooner you incorporate Clean Eating in your household the sooner your children will also adopt Clean Eating habits and become healthier and slimmer. It is your job to set the example as it is with everything. Kids won't suspect you are literally saving their lives if you serve them grilled chicken, brown rice, fresh fruit and vegetables, or a bowl of steaming oatmeal. However, you will soon notice your child losing excess fat and getting brighter, clearer skin. You will also notice improved overall health, improved mood and improved brain power. It's worth it for you and your entire family. You are holding the opportunity to change your kids' lives and yours in your hands by nature of this book. You'll be handing your children an outstanding set of survival tools that will serve them well throughout their adult lives.

BE INFORMED

www.cdc.gov/nccdphp/dnpa/obesity
www.hc-sc.gc.ca/iyh-vsv/life-vie/obes_e.html
www.activehealthykids.ca
www.keepkidshealthy.com
www.nedic.ca
www.nationaleatingdisorders.org

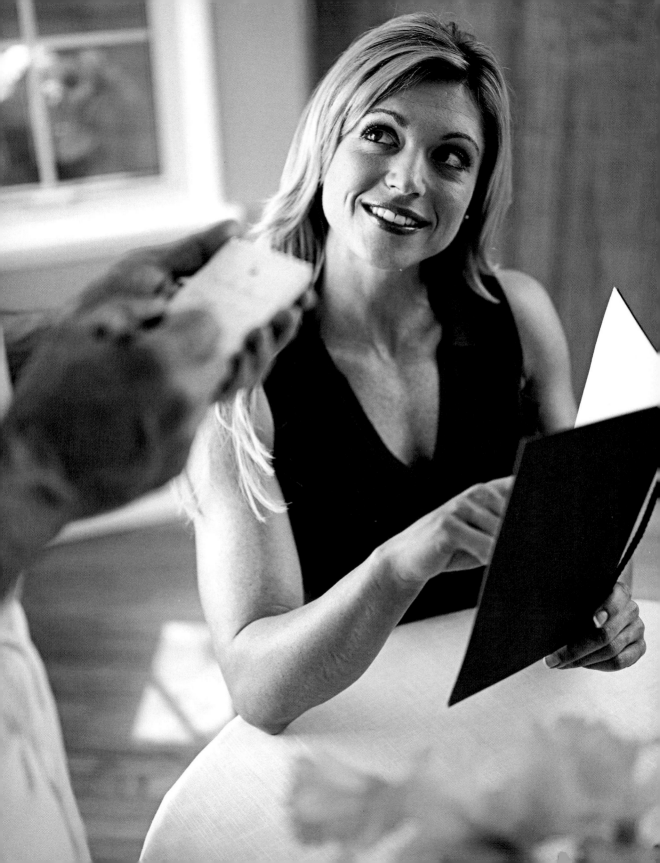

CHAPTER NINE

ORDERING
OUT

BILLIONS ON THE TABLE

It is far less expensive and far better for your Clean-Eating aspirations to cook at home, but there will be times when you will not be able to avoid eating out. Statistics prove it. In the United States alone, each year an estimated $400 billion is spent for food prepared somewhere other than at home – either in restaurants or take-out stands. In the past few decades dining out has been the most noticeable change in North American eating habits. The problem with this trend is that foods consumed away from home contain more poor-quality nutrients, including saturated and trans fats, than those consumed at home. Those same foods contain more sodium and sugar and less calcium and fiber.

In the past dining out was an occasional treat. Today dining out is no longer occasional. People probably do not realize to what extent dining out has become part of the North American way of life, either financially or calorically. Since the trend for dining out doesn't show any signs of slowing, it is exceedingly important to give your dining experience careful thought. It is both possible and trouble-free to Eat Clean while eating out, as long as you have a game plan on how to accomplish it.

WHAT IS YOUR MINDSET?

Usually a trip to a restaurant is synonymous with celebration, relaxation or reward. Most restaurant patrons don't consider the nutritional quality of foods they eat in a restaurant in the same way they do foods eaten at home. Dining out is partnered with the attitude of taking a break, and since you are paying a premium for "restaurant food" you are less willing to sacrifice taste. With temptation being on the menu tonight, it's likely to be a challenge for you to get through it and order clean foods successfully. Will you cave in when you see the menu or will you stick to the plan? Presumably you have read the previous chapters and tried at least some of the Clean-Eating principles, so it would be counter-productive to blow your hard work now.

ORDER CLEAN AND EAT CLEAN

No matter what restaurant you plan to visit, from a five-star resort to a diner, it is possible to order and Eat Clean. I always approach eating out with a review of my physique goals. If I am in the middle of preparing for a particular goal, I make every effort to

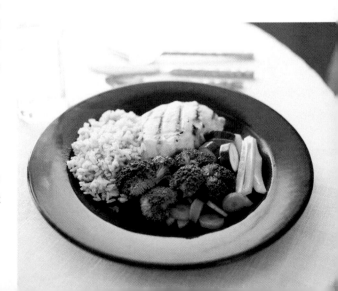

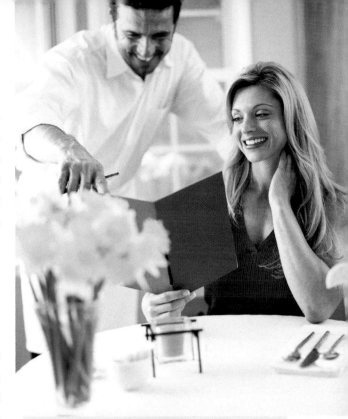

keep myself within the tightest limits of Clean Eating. I won't eat bread, order a glass of wine or eat dessert. If you've recently lost a few pounds and want to keep on losing weight, you'll stay strict too. Some of you may just have started Eating Clean and there are others of you who are maintaining a Clean Eating lifestyle. Ultimately you will have to determine where you are in the process and order accordingly.

MAKE FRIENDS WITH THE SERVER

The best piece of advice I can give you when ordering clean in a restaurant is to make friends with your server. Without the server on your side you will never get the clean food you want. It's helpful to your plan to let your server know you are interested in ordering but that you want your food prepared without added sauces, gravies, butters, fats and oils. Use your charm in a firm but polite manner to win him or her over. Keep your instructions simple. Once you have charmed him into your corner, tell him politely but meaningfully that you will return the food if it comes covered in the things you didn't want.

ORDERING FROM THE MENU

No matter what your goals, it's time to incorporate your Clean-Eating habits into the dining out experience. Let's scan the menu. Tonight the chef's feature item is salmon with a maple syrup glaze. Most people

Let your server know you are interested in ordering but that you want your food prepared without added sauces, gravies, butters, fats and oils.

would order the salmon as it comes, never daring to request a different preparation. But that is exactly what you are going to do. Order the salmon but tell the server you want it "dry." Sometimes you have to make sure the server understands your request so it helps to repeat the request in a friendly way. Once you make friends with the server and explain you want your food prepared a little differently, it is a simple matter to get your food the way you want it. If you are running into resistance, suggest you are avoiding certain food items because they make you sick or you are allergic. Don't worry about the chef in the kitchen either. It is not beyond his or her capabilities to prepare the fish without a sauce.

Let's move on to the vegetables. The broccoli and cauliflower accompanying the salmon are served with a heavy cream and cheese sauce. You definitely don't want either the sauce or the load of calories and fat in this mixture. Once again, ask the server to serve your vegetables without sauce. Request steamed vegetables instead. Often vegetables are served with melted butter. You'll have to anticipate this too and request your veggies plain. Tell the server you will send the order back if there is any sauce or butter on your food. If you ask firmly but politely, and with a smile, you'll have no trouble.

Should the fish and vegetables come with brown rice, order it, but this is rare unless you're in a savvy restaurant. You can ask to switch the accompanying starch, whether it's some form of potato, rice or noodle, to an extra helping of vegetables if you are really keeping your food intake tight. If I am dining

late I often omit starchy carbohydrates because I know I will not be able to burn off the added calories. Appetizers are a minefield of extra calories if you are not careful. Onion soup has a thick layer of melted cheese on top of it and the broth is often greasy. If you are interested in soup for a starter, make sure to check with the server to find out whether it is broth or cream based. Puréed vegetable soups are a delicious source of complex carbohydrates and nutrients but you don't want to kill the effect of that if the soup is made with cream. Ask the server to be sure. If there are no Clean-Eating appetizer choices, ask for a salad instead. Remember, bacon bits and croutons are not on your Clean-Eating menu, so make sure they are not on your salad. Dress the salad with lemon juice or balsamic vinegar and olive oil. Herbs are fine. Chilled shrimp cocktail with lemon is a good choice too.

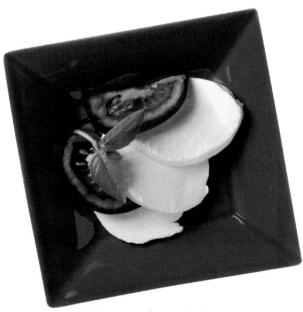

If the breadbasket is too tempting to avoid, ask the waiter not to bring it at all. Placing a basket of bread on the table is a ploy used by restaurant owners to keep the customers happy and full while entrées and appetizers are being prepared. But having a fragrant basket of bread sitting under your nose makes your job of resisting much more difficult. Fill up on water and enjoy your companions' conversation but omit the bread.

THAT COULD FEED FOUR OF US!

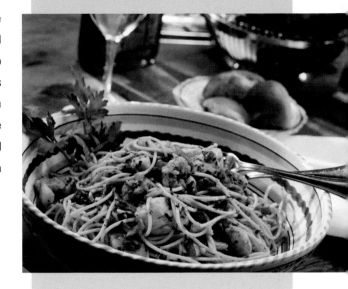

North American restaurants are famed for serving enormous portions. Quantities are often so large they could feed more than one person. This coincides with findings from a study wherein the average daily caloric intake in 1955 was 1807 but rose to 2043 calories per day in 1987-88. At the same time the CDC reports that one in three adults is overweight. Some of the increase in calories consumed is definitely because of the number of meals eaten in restaurants. According to **Biing-Hwan Lin, Joanne Guthrie and Elizabeth Frazao**, authors of a report entitled *Nutrient Contribution of Food Away from Home*, "…when eating out, people either eat more food or eat higher-calorie foods – or both."

It is up to you to control your food intake. Keep the Clean-Eating-recommended portion sizes in your mind and consider whether or not the salad you just ordered at The Cheesecake Factory will feed you or the four of you for lunch. Remember the protein

"**…when eating out, people either eat more food or eat higher-calorie foods – or both.**"

serving should approximate the size of the palm of your hand, complex carbohydrates from fresh vegetables the size of two hands cupped together and whole grains the size of one cupped hand. Consider ordering a starter for a main course if the restaurant you are in has a reputation for serving large portions. Also consider that at home you may not eat an appetizer while in a restaurant situation you might. That means you will be eating more and taking in more calories so you'll have to adjust your food intake accordingly if you want to stick to Clean Eating.

DOGGIE BAG PLEASE!

Just because you have received an enormous portion of food on your plate doesn't mean you must finish all of it. You can ask for a doggie bag right away and put half of the food away or you can doggie-bag it afterwards. Regardless, you are not obligated to wolf it all down. You are the one paying for this food, so taking the extra home is your right. And believe me – restaurants do not mind this at all and it happens all the time, so don't be embarrassed. Just be sure to remember it when you leave!

"When it comes to birthday cake, I will take a very small piece but won't eat the icing or ice cream."

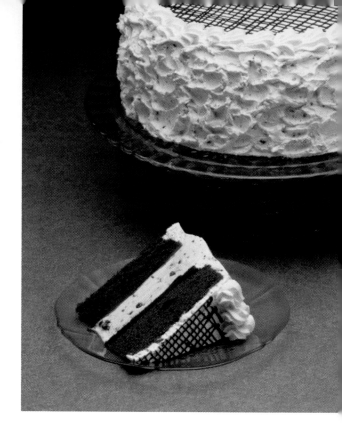

DESSERT IS STICKY!

Dessert can be sticky. The general offerings on a dessert menu are definitely not geared towards Clean Eating. Unfortunately people do love dessert – they really are treats. Few of us can resist fragrant apple pie served with ice cream, crème brulée, chocolate cake and a host of decadent meal finishers. What birthday is complete without birthday cake? Once again, when it comes to ordering dessert you will have to ask yourself where you stand in your goals. I usually keep my dessert eating to a few limited occasions, including birthdays, holidays like Christmas or Thanksgiving and the odd very special celebration. Even then that's about 20 desserts per year and that's more than enough for me. If I am hosting the meal for Christmas and Thanksgiving –

and I usually do because I have the biggest dining room table — I always prepare Clean-Eating dessert choices. The simplest ones are fruit salads, fresh berry combinations, fruit platters and unsweetened applesauce. I occasionally make biscotti since they are naturally low in fat and calories and I have a special oatmeal cookie recipe (on page 249) that wins rave reviews at every family feast. When it comes to birthday cake, I will take a very small piece but won't eat the icing and ask for no ice cream.

In a restaurant I will ask the server if there are fresh berries or a selection of fresh fruits for dessert. I don't always order dessert but if I want it and have decided I can afford the added calories, fresh fruit or berries is what I will have. In some ways it's bold of me to ask, especially when what I am asking for is not on the menu, but I do it anyway because I see berries used as garnish on someone else's dessert or in a beverage. There's no harm in asking and you'd be amazed what comes to the table sometimes. I have yet to be disappointed.

ALCOHOL — DESSERT OR DRINK?

Alcohol is another form of sugar with as many unnecessary calories from sugar as a dessert. It's dessert poured into a glass rather than being served on a plate — whether or not that alcohol actually tastes sweet. Sugar is a bogey when it comes to Clean Eating. Specialty liqueurs like Bailey's Irish Cream or Kahlua are delicious but absolutely thick with sugar. Such beverages don't come with nutrition labels, but they include hefty doses of sugar; definitely not on your Clean-Eating list of recommend foods. In general it is best to avoid or limit alcohol intake.

If you must have a little something, drink one glass of dry red wine or have a spritzer — that's white wine mixed with soda water. Ask for the diet ginger ale! Unless a lot of people are going to drink wine with me at the dinner table, I usually order by the glass. That way I won't feel obliged to finish the whole bottle.

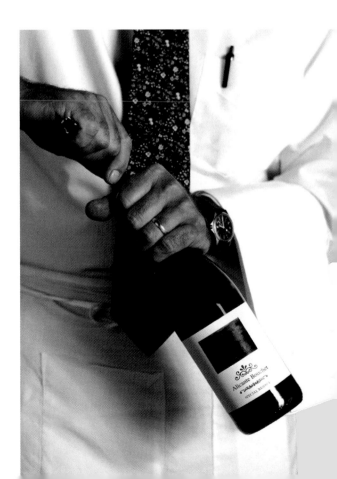

WAITER, YOU GOT THAT WRONG!

There will be times, more frequent than you would like, when the chef or the server gets your order wrong. If your Clean-Eating requests were ignored and your entrée comes to you swimming in cheese sauce while the accompanying potato is crowned with a blob of sour cream, you have a problem. What do you do?

Don't wimp out now! You've been with me all along reading this book, shopping and Eating Clean and making amazing progress. You've worked hard to lose a few pounds. I don't want you to cave in out of fear or complacency. Stick with your resolve to Eat Clean. Remind the server that you ordered your meal without accoutrement and would like it that way. The wait staff will usually be happy to oblige you by going back to the kitchen and cleaning up your order. If you run into a problem, make a mental note not to go to that restaurant again.

IT GETS EASIER

I eat out frequently when I travel so I have to handle the dining-out situation a lot. I have found that most chefs are fairly accommodating if you are polite. They are chefs after all and love their craft. As reported by **Biing-Hwan Lin, Joanne Guthrie** and **Elizabeth Frazao** in *Nutrient Contribution of Food Away from Home*, "There is no intrinsic reason why food away from home must differ nutritionally from food prepared at home. Indeed, professional chefs and foodservice organizations may be particularly adept at preparing good-tasting meals that meet dietary recommendations." I am not afraid to order my food clean since I am the one paying and want to eat properly all the time.

MAKING A COMMITMENT TO YOURSELF

Your current physique pretty much reflects what you are putting into it. The body doesn't lie. It tells the truth. If you are neglecting both nutrition and exercise you'll look, well, soft and squishy, a lot like the donuts you love to eat. If you enjoy eating, can't locate the OFF button, and on top of that have no inclination to exercise, then you'll look like the couch you're lying on – softer and squishier.

On the other hand, if you show equal respect for both nutrition and exercise, your body becomes a reflection of your discipline. Skin, hair, eyes and nails glow with health. Muscles ripple under tight skin. Your waist is trim and your heart beats at a steady, moderate pace. There is no excess flesh anywhere.

When people complain to me that they are doing everything but are still fat, I know the body doesn't lie. Those folks are getting something wrong and 95 percent of the time it's either what, or how much, they are shoveling into their mouths. Let your physique paint an accurate picture of what you are doing. Eating Clean is the best and only way to accomplish that.

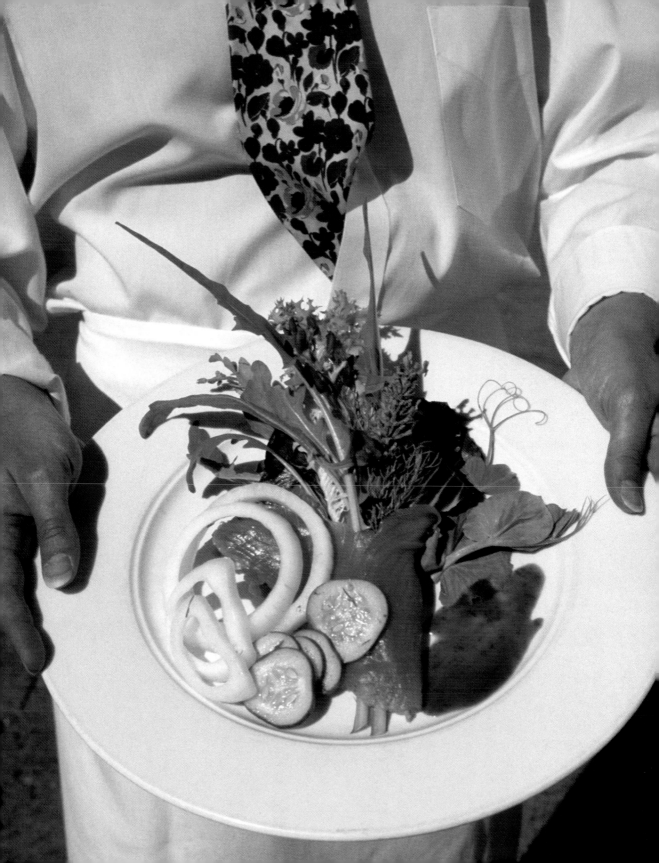

CAN I GET THAT GRILLED?

Here are several techniques to help you with your Clean-Eating ordering. Stay committed to your plan, not only to improve your nutrition but also your health. Weight loss will be the ultimate result. Good for you!

- **Take the breadbasket away.** The bread is on the table to keep you busy while your meal is being prepared.

- **Substitute** vegetables, including salad greens and sliced tomatoes, for fries.

- **Drink your coffee black or with skim milk.**

- **Have your protein grilled, baked, steamed or poached.** These cooking techniques reduce unnecessary fat in your meal.

- **Try sushi or sashimi** from a reputable source as a great Clean-Eating protein alternative.

- **Order an appetizer as an entrée** if you aren't overly hungry.

- **Ask for a doggie bag** right away if the portion is too large.

- *"Waiter, is that cream in my soup?"* **Ask the server if a food item is prepared with cream, butter or other high-calorie ingredients.** Don't order the entrée if you aren't sure.

- **Ask for dressings and sauces to be served on the side.** Balsamic vinegar and mustard rule!

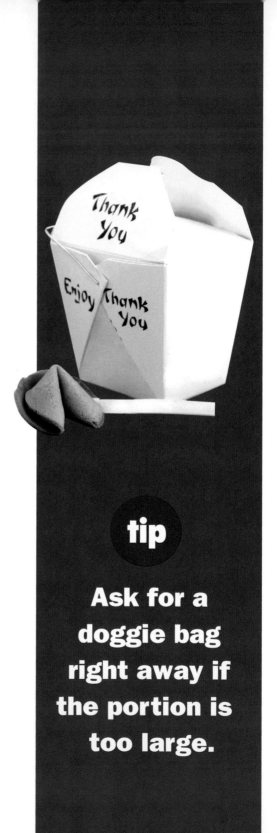

tip

Ask for a doggie bag right away if the portion is too large.

MENU TRANSLATIONS

Take a few minutes to study the menu before placing your order. Ordering too hastily could result in a disappointing meal loaded with **unnecessary fats, sodium and sugar.**

HIGH-CALORIE TRAP	TRANSLATION
Au gratin	With cheese
Basted	To moisten meat with fat or drippings
Battered	A fat, flour and water mixture to coat meat
Béarnaise	Cream sauce of egg yolks, vinegar and butter
Béchamel	Cream sauce of milk, butter and flour
Bisque	Shellfish purée of wine, cognac and fresh cream
Breaded	Coated with mixture of breadcrumbs, egg & butter
Buttered	Butter added to the dish
Creamed/creamy	Cream added to the dish
Crisp (savory)	Fried in butter or oil
Crisp (sweet)	Topping of butter and sugar
Croquette	Mixture of meat or grains bound w/ heavy sauce & deep fried
Croute	Encased in pastry and fried in butter
Custard	Sweet sauce of eggs, cream, milk, butter & sugar
Foie gras	Duck or goose liver
Fried, fritters, frite	Anything fried in oil
Hollandaise	Hot sauce of egg yolks and butter
Parmesan	With parmesan cheese
Scalloped	Layered dish of vegetables & sauce made of milk, butter & flour
Tempura	Batter coating of ice water, flour and eggs, fried

CLEAN EATING TERM ➔	TRANSLATION
Au jus	In its own juice
Baked	Oven cooked, no added oils, fats or sauce
Braised	Slow cooked in its own juice
Broiled	Cooked under high heat
Ceviche	Raw fish, citrus juice, limes, onion and tomato
Gazpacho	Spanish uncooked soup made with tomato, cucumber, onion, red pepper, olive oil, corn & spices
Grilled	Cooked over high heat to seal in natural juices
Lean	Without added fat
Poached	Simmered in liquid
Purée	Blended foods
Roasted	Cooking foods in radiant heat of oven or over open flame
Salsa	Spicy sauce of uncooked vegetables or fruit, usually tomatoes, onions, peppers and herbs
Sauté	Cook meat, vegetables or fish in very small amount of fat in frying pan until brown
Steamed	Foods cooked over but not in boiling water

"Professional chefs and foodservice organizations may be particularly adept at preparing good-tasting meals that meet dietary recommendations."

Biing-Hwan Lin, Joanne Guthrie and Elizabeth Frazao in **Nutrient Contribution of Food Away from Home**

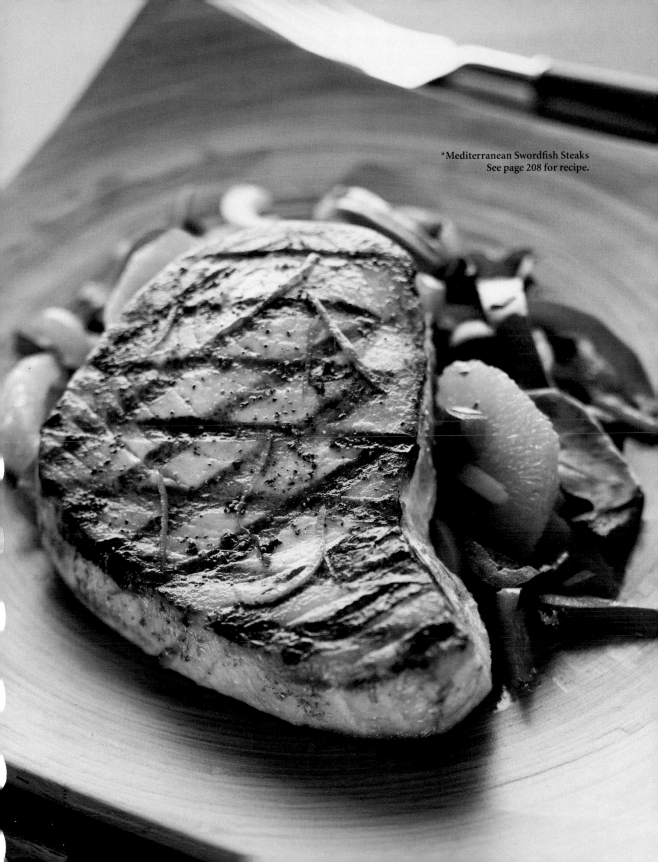

*Mediterranean Swordfish Steaks
See page 208 for recipe.

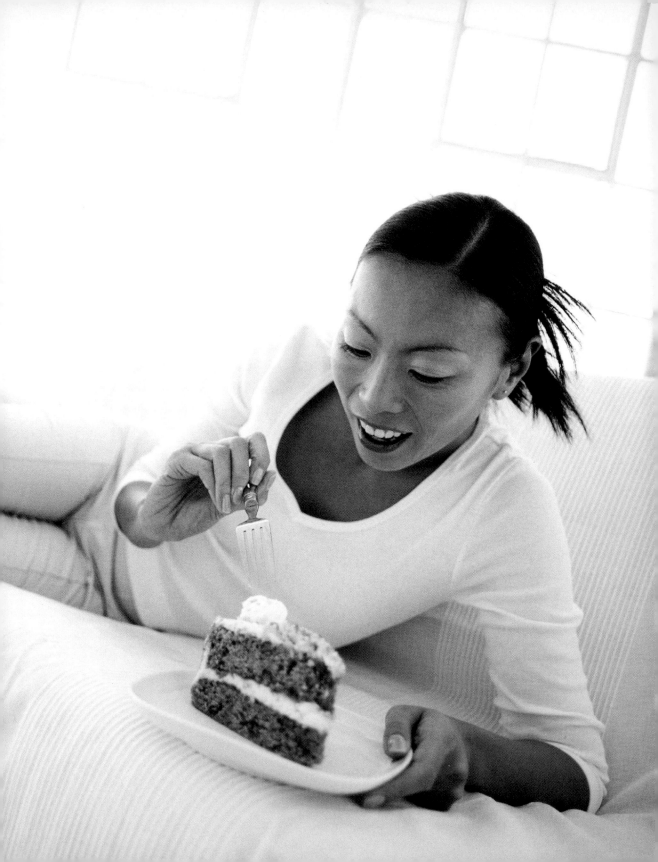

CHAPTER TEN

CHEATING

A LEARNING EXPERIENCE

MAKING A DEAL

One of the most difficult decisions you can make is the one to go on a diet. Tougher still is staying on it. By the time you've decided to do it, you want the weight to have been lost yesterday. So you make a deal with yourself, leaving no room for error. You begin by telling yourself there will be no cheating, no eating and no repeating of past mistakes. And then one day … you eat a chocolate bar. But it doesn't stop there. Now you've messed up your diet anyway, you might as well have a frothy carb-loaded concoction. So you get really depressed and dive into a tub of ice cream. In the end, results are often slim to none and short-lived.

I know. I've made similar promises to myself before I started Eating Clean. Everyone does. Eating Clean changed everything for me.

One of the most difficult decisions you can make is the one to go on a diet. Tougher still is staying on it.

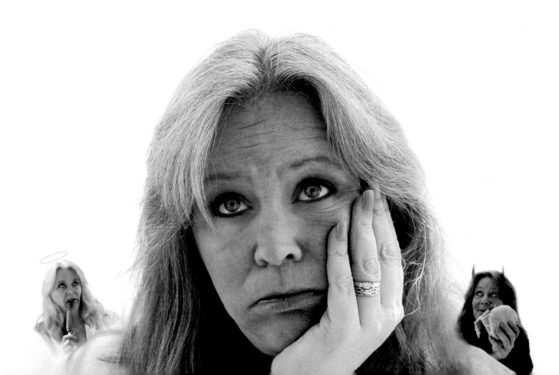

DO YOU KNOW SOMEONE LIKE THIS?

I wonder if you know someone like the woman in this story. I have a friend who swears she Eats Clean. "Really!" she'll insist. She is currently more than 30 pounds overweight but she claims she keeps her diet tight. "Oh, I never eat cookies or ice cream. I just Eat Clean but no matter what I do or don't eat, I'm still overweight." She'll sigh heavily at the end of her sad tale and look at me hopefully. I suppose she's wondering if there's some way I can fix it. You know what her husband told me? He said he knew why his wife was overweight. He loves to putter in his garden. Often when he's been outdoors poking about in his beloved flowers he's caught a glimpse of his wife in the kitchen. There he would see her sawing off a great hunk of cheese and cramming it in her mouth. It wasn't that he spied on her. He just caught her doing it so often. This disturbed him and so he'd quickly turn away. It turns out she has been sneaking food all this time.

I receive stacks of letters and e-mails from *Oxygen* readers like this who hope I can help them fix their problem. I can't, but they will find if they truly do Eat Clean their own bodies will help them.

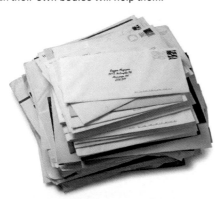

WHAT I KNOW

Here's something I do know for sure. Clean Eating works so well and so consistently, there is no possible way you can gain weight following this lifestyle. How do I know? I've done it for several years. My weight never varies more than a few pounds, and those pounds inevitably creep up when I don't Eat Clean. I'll be traveling somewhere or it will be one of my daughter's birthdays and I'll relent just a little. I'll have a wedge of cake just to be sociable, then I'll have a slice of bread when I wouldn't normally and pretty soon I've gained three pounds. It happens that quickly. I would not be surprised if it happened that fast for you too. I'm very in tune with my body so I know right away when I've gone too far off the rails. Not only do the scales tell me, my clothes tell me.

The Eat-Clean Diet is the only book that deals with cheating head on. Entire books are written about what to eat, what not to eat and when to eat it but not a single one helps you overcome the obstacle everyone faces but no one wants to admit.

YOU'RE TEMPTED

Everyone gets tempted. Everyone cheats when on a diet. It's not the same as cheating on a math exam. What are the consequences when you stray from a diet? You don't get a failing grade. You have to answer only to yourself. It's human to weaken and it's human to want to "reward" yourself. That's how many of us view cheating; as an opportunity to pat ourselves on the back because we've been so good. You might say, "I just couldn't help myself!" when faced with a bowl of your favorite ice cream. And let's not forget about giving in to Mom's oatmeal chocolate chip cookies and buttery, gravy-laden mashed potatoes.

GIVING UP

When I decided to win my life and my body back I had to abandon several sources of temptation. I love cheese and still do – I'm Dutch after all. I suppose I was born with the gene of loving cheese. Then there's peanut butter and ice cream. These are my favorites and none of them qualify as Clean-Eating foods.

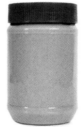

Cheese contains anywhere from 35 to 60 percent fat, so that had to go. Sometimes I'll have a piece of reduced-fat cheese but it just doesn't taste the same so I normally don't bother. Commercial peanut butter contains 76 percent fat, some hydrogenated, and added sugar. Ughhh! I can just hear the fat collecting on my hips and thighs. I had to give that up too but I found a Clean-Eating alternative in the form of natural nut butters, including peanut, cashew, almond and a variety of others. You need good fats in your diet and these nut butters are delicious, so I'm happy with them. As for ice cream, I relegate it to very special occasions only. It's just too tempting. I don't buy it, because no matter where I stash it in the freezer, I'll find it later.

CHEATING IS LEARNING

I learned to regard cheating as part of the lifestyle renovation I was working on. Believe it or not, cheating serves a purpose. Once you've indulged in your particular brand of sin, the pleasure is short-lived. The treats taste good while you're indulging but soon afterwards you feel as if you've made a big mistake. Think about the hard work you accomplished in the last week; the hours on the treadmill, 42 Clean-Eating meals prepared and enjoyed and hundreds of pounds of weights pushed and pulled in the gym. Is one bowl of ice cream going to take you down? What if you've cheated for an entire day or, heaven forbid, an entire weekend? Even so, the object of your focus remains the same. Put the cheating behind you. You still want to make significant weight-loss improvements, so let the cheating serve as your motivation to tighten up today.

The treats taste good while you're indulging but soon afterwards you feel as if you've made a big mistake.

When I've had a glass of wine or a day of less-than-Clean Eating I don't let it get me down. I use it to motivate me back in the direction I was heading – toward a lean, toned body. I realize that some of you want to give up entirely when you step off the rails, saying, "No diet

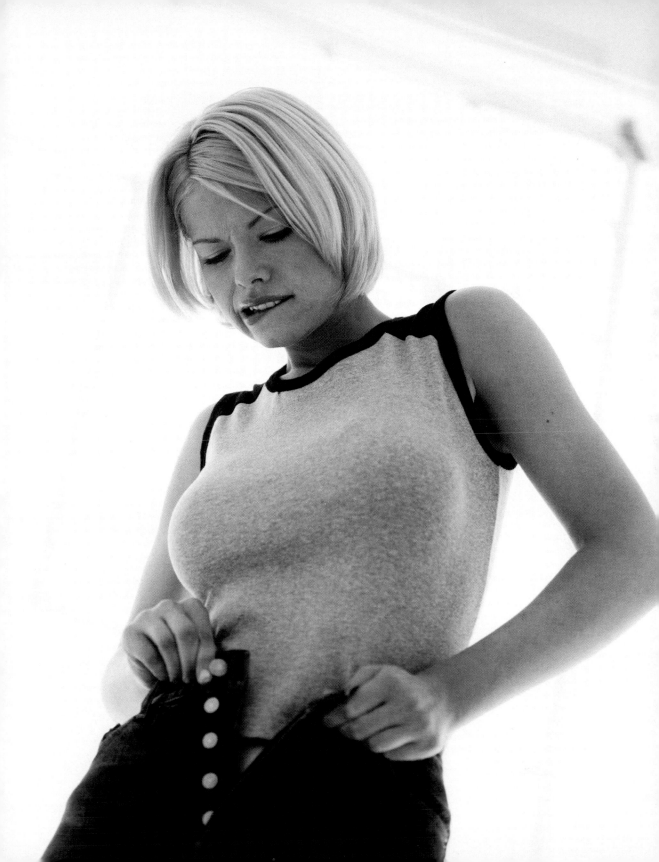

works for me!" That's how yo-yo dieting happens. Clean Eating helps you get back on track.

MAKE A PLAN

You need a plan at the ready so when temptation arises you'll be prepared. Think about the piece of birthday cake that may face you at the office. Ask yourself how badly you want it. Decide if the cake is more immediate than your desire to Eat Clean with the ultimate reward of a gorgeous physique. And let's not forget the hard work you've pumped into your training. By now you'll know what your answer will be. The answer depends on you and your resolution towards cheating and treating. Know your limits.

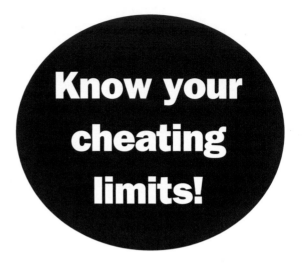

Know your cheating limits!

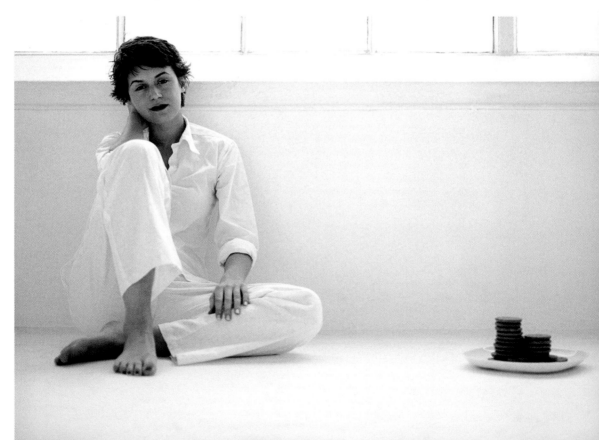

Some men plan a full day of cheating. Everything they eat is garbage but they don't care. It makes them "feel better." They put it on their weekly schedule just as they slot in leg training or cardio. Women, on the other hand, don't usually enjoy an entire day of cheating once they've started Eating Clean. They don't want to waste their hard-won results. Some of my gym friends have a latte once in a while, but that is the end of it. Others splurge with pizza or ice cream every once in a while. The extra calories from one cheat meal or treat are a lot easier to burn off than several hundred – or even thousand – from an entire day of overindulgence.

Eating Clean is a healthy lifestyle. Bingeing for an entire day isn't. Bingeing, cheating, over-indulging … none of these belong in the Clean-Eating healthy lifestyle. Everything about Clean Eating is positive and builds self-esteem. Every rep you take with weights builds a strong body and mind. Every step you take as you run or walk, liberates you from that former flabby self. You're on your way to a glorious new one. Many *Oxygen* readers write to me saying Eating Clean has saved their lives. They no longer suffer from chronic pain, irritable bowel syndrome, constipation, hypoglycemia, mood swings and a host of other conditions.

I prefer to think of cheating as treating. Slot yourself in for one treat a week. Have a cookie with your latte. Enjoy! But that's it for that week.

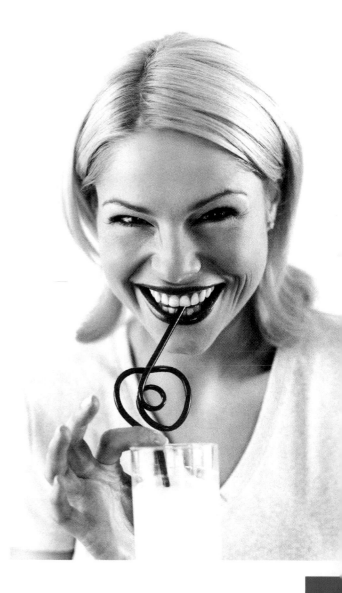

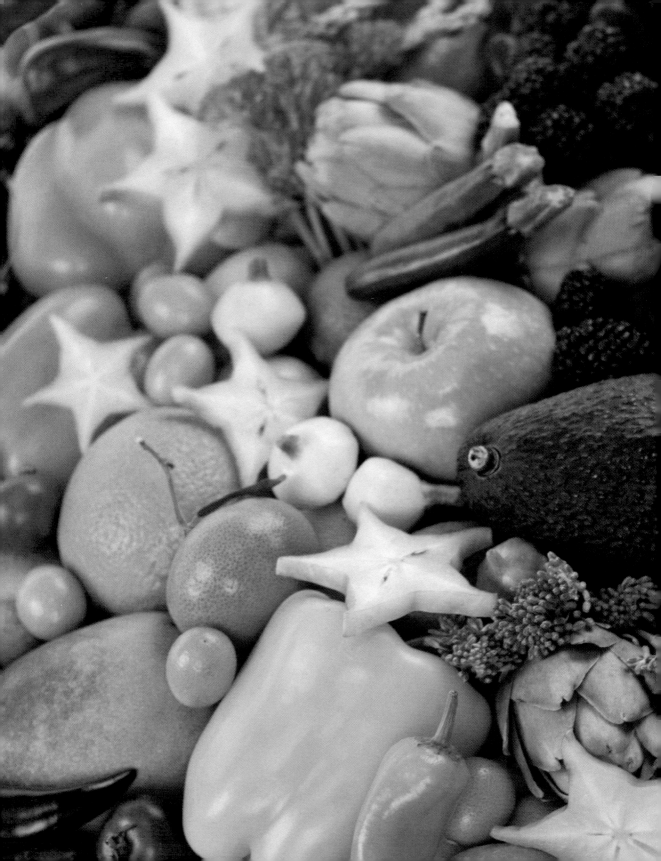

CHAPTER ELEVEN

SUPPLEMENTS & SUPERFOODS

Supplements are a lot like manure and mulch in your garden. You don't really need them but when you use them these fertilizers make plants grow better, healthier, stronger and more able to resist disease. If you can accomplish that for yourself with a bit of human fertilizer, namely supplements, why wouldn't you? The human version of manure and mulch or fertilizer comes in the form of vitamins, protein supplements, and superfoods. You don't purchase these at the hardware store but you can find them virtually anywhere else.

It can be enormously disconcerting to try and sort out which supplements to take. There are thousands of different kinds and so many brands. Where does a person begin to make sense of this profusion? Every day there's yet another supplement you should take for its life-saving qualities. It's understandable that you may be confused. I was until I thoroughly researched this vast category of supplements over the years. I made it my business to investigate supplements, and I did it by reading all the materials I could get my hands on and trying some out. I came to realize Eating Clean is a way of supplementing your nutrition, because the basis of the lifestyle depends on nourishing the body with wholesome, natural foods. You will feel and look better eating this way and using these superfoods and supplements.

WHAT IS A SUPPLEMENT?

A supplement by definition is an ingredient added to complete a thing, make up a deficiency, or extend or strengthen the whole. Vitamins, minerals, enzymes, supplements and superfoods all make up for nutritional deficiencies.

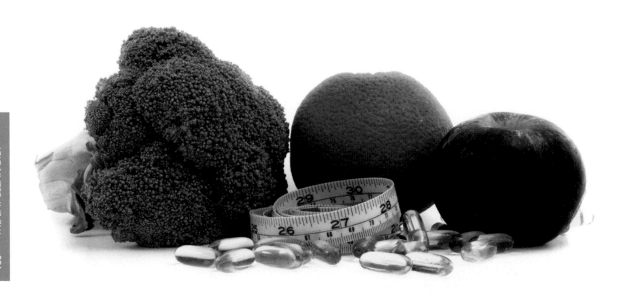

SUPERFOODS

Superfoods are supplements, but not the kind you are used to. In the days of our parents and theirs, no one talked about "superfoods," because people routinely ate oatmeal, broccoli, salmon, nuts, flaxseed and milk – foods densely charged with nutritional elements. If you currently eat loads of refined carbohydrates, adding fresh fruits and vegetables supplements the lesser ingredients. When Clean Eating becomes routine for you, you may not need to be reminded to eat tomatoes any longer, but until then, consider fresh produce, whole grains, legumes and lean meats your supplemental superfoods. If you already eat broccoli and carrots, good for you, but consider adding a few more items from the Clean-Eating Superfoods and Supplements lists.

LET'S SORT IT OUT

It is easy to believe in a magic pill that promises stunning weight loss and glowing health. North American society likes to believe in such things. In reality, of course, nothing of that nature exists. No pill guarantees that kind of success in a healthy manner. Clean Eating can guarantee weight loss in a healthy way because it is accomplished by eating wholesome natural foods low in added fats, salt and sugars. Not only is Clean Eating healthy, it is long term. However, there are some supplements and superfoods you should add to your nutrition in order to get their complete healthful benefits.

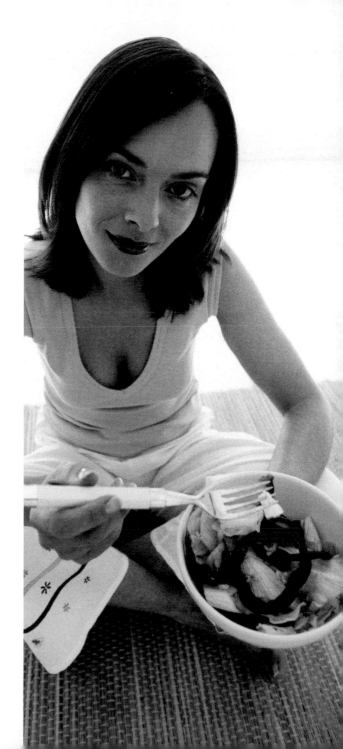

SUPERFOODS
FOR YOU

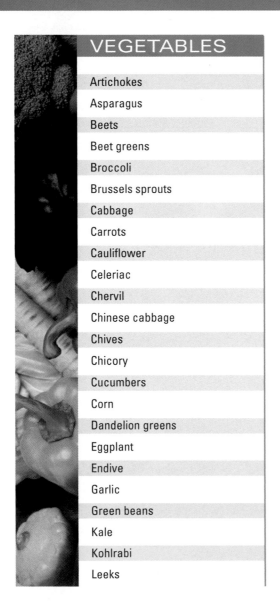

VEGETABLES

Artichokes

Asparagus

Beets

Beet greens

Broccoli

Brussels sprouts

Cabbage

Carrots

Cauliflower

Celeriac

Chervil

Chinese cabbage

Chives

Chicory

Cucumbers

Corn

Dandelion greens

Eggplant

Endive

Garlic

Green beans

Kale

Kohlrabi

Leeks

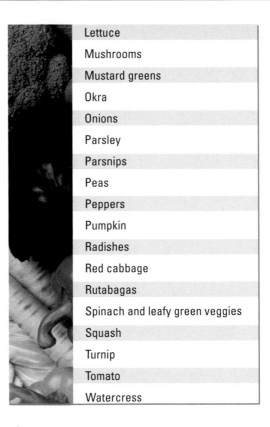

Lettuce

Mushrooms

Mustard greens

Okra

Onions

Parsley

Parsnips

Peas

Peppers

Pumpkin

Radishes

Red cabbage

Rutabagas

Spinach and leafy green veggies

Squash

Turnip

Tomato

Watercress

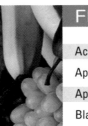

FRUITS

Acai and goji berries

Apples

Apricots

Blackberries

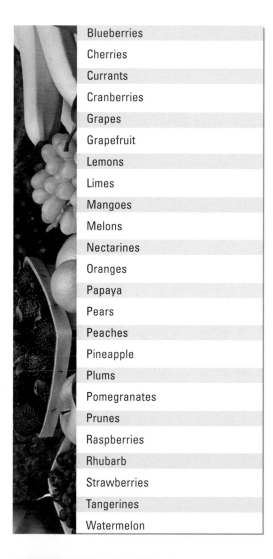

Blueberries
Cherries
Currants
Cranberries
Grapes
Grapefruit
Lemons
Limes
Mangoes
Melons
Nectarines
Oranges
Papaya
Pears
Peaches
Pineapple
Plums
Pomegranates
Prunes
Raspberries
Rhubarb
Strawberries
Tangerines
Watermelon

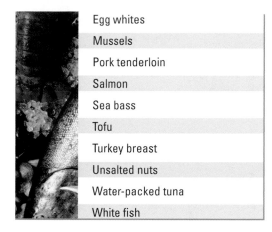

Egg whites
Mussels
Pork tenderloin
Salmon
Sea bass
Tofu
Turkey breast
Unsalted nuts
Water-packed tuna
White fish

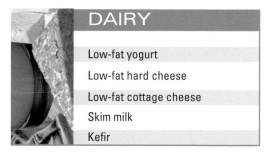

DAIRY

Low-fat yogurt
Low-fat hard cheese
Low-fat cottage cheese
Skim milk
Kefir

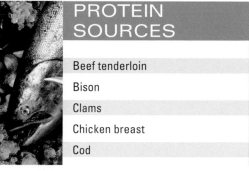

PROTEIN SOURCES

Beef tenderloin
Bison
Clams
Chicken breast
Cod

Keep this list handy while grocery shopping.

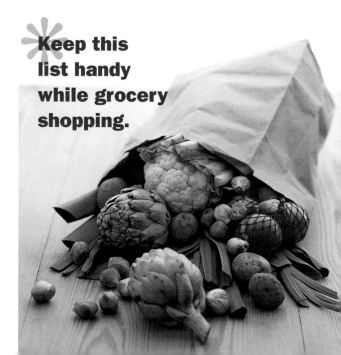

TOP **12** SUPERFOODS

1 TOMATO

It's not a vegetable, it's actually a fruit. Tomatoes are one of the most popular superfoods and an ideal Clean-Eating food. They are enjoyed both fresh and cooked year-round in a variety of foods. Phytochemicals in their ripe red flesh prevent free radicals from damaging joints, muscles and brain cells. It is easier for the body to assimilate lycopene, the tomato's potent phytochemical, once it has been cooked, but tomatoes are delicious cooked or fresh.

HINT: Winter tomatoes often taste dreadful. Try roasting them in the oven to improve their flavor. Simply wash plum tomatoes. Halve them and lay them flat on a nonstick cookie sheet. Roast at 350°F for 25 minutes. Enjoy!

STORAGE TIPS: Don't store fresh tomatoes in the fridge or with other fruits. Ripening tomatoes emit a gas that causes other fruits in proximity to rot. Place tomatoes in a bowl on the counter where they will ripen. This helps their flavor improve.

✳ STAR NUTRIENTS:

- ✳ Lycopene for fighting cancer, especially prostate cancer.
- ✳ Carotenoids, especially beta-carotene, a powerful antioxidant.

NUTRIENTS PER HALF-CUP SERVING:

Calories:	17
Protein:	1 g
Fiber:	1 g
Potassium:	250 mg
Beta carotene:	620 mcg
Vitamin C:	17 mg
Vitamin E:	1 mg
Folate:	17 mcg

SKINLESS TURKEY BREAST 2

White-meat turkey breast without the skin is often overlooked because it is considered a special-occasion food – think Thanksgiving or Christmas. Turkey is a superfood because it is nutrient-dense yet low in calories. Turkey is supercharged, loaded with lean protein, vitamins, and minerals and that makes it suitable to include in your Clean-Eating lifestyle. Substitute turkey for red meat often. Use lean ground turkey breast in place of ground beef.

✳ Lean protein

✳ Minerals

NUTRIENTS PER SIX-OUNCE SERVING:

Calories:	230
Protein:	51 g
Cholesterol:	142 mg
Sodium:	90 mg
Potassium:	699 mcg
Calcium:	5 mg

ALSO CONTAINS
- **Niacin**
- **Vitamin B6**
- **Vitamin B12**
- **Iron**
- **Selenium**
- **Zinc**

FACT: SEDENTARY ADULT WOMEN REQUIRE 46 GRAMS OF PROTEIN PER DAY. WOMEN TRAINING WITH WEIGHTS REQUIRE 56 GRAMS OF PROTEIN OR MORE EACH DAY. WOMEN TRYING TO GROW MUSCLE SHOULD EAT ONE GRAM OF PROTEIN PER POUND OF BODYWEIGHT PER DAY.

TIP: Turkey and chicken breast meat contain the phytochemical carnosine. This compound preserves muscle and brain tissue. Carnosine is often given to performance athletes to improve endurance and muscle formation.

WILD SALMON   3

Wild salmon contains fewer growth hormones and toxins than its farm-raised cousin. Wild salmon is a nutrient-dense source of quality, easily digested protein, vitamins, and minerals, and is low in saturated fat. The fats found in this fish are highly specialized EFAs, or essential fatty acids, necessary for keeping body tissue healthy and free from inflammation. Try to include more servings of fish in your Clean-Eating menu.

✳ STAR NUTRIENTS:

✳ Protein

✳ Essential fatty acids

NUTRIENTS PER THREE-OUNCE SERVING:

Calories:	155
Protein:	22 g
Sodium:	48 mg
Essential fatty acids:	6.9 g

ALSO CONTAINS
- **Vitamin D**
- **Marine omega-3 fatty acids**
- **Vitamin B**
- **Selenium**

TONING FACTOR:

The flesh of wild salmon contains a powerful antioxidant – DMAE, or dimethylaminoethanol – which stimulates nerve function and tones muscle. Recently it has shown up in facial creams, where it is said to "lift" sagging, wrinkled skin. DMAE also helps improve memory function.

WILD IS RED:

Ask for wild fish at your local fish counter. You'll know you're getting wild when you see the intense red flesh. Farmed salmon is usually much lighter in color.

4 BROCCOLI

Broccoli happens to be one of the best-selling vegetables in North America. Its crunchy, albeit smelly, cousins – kale, cabbage, turnip, cauliflower and Brussels sprouts – are equally well stocked with disease-fighting nutrients. These stinky greens are known to boost the immune system by fortifying it with a cancer-fighting phytochemical called sulforaphane. Broccoli is a nutritional superfood. One serving contains more vitamin C than a glass of orange juice. Broccoli can be used in Clean-Eating menus from breakfast through to supper.

✳ STAR NUTRIENTS:

✳ Folate

✳ Vitamin C

Calories:	33
Iron:	2 mg
Folate:	90 mcg
Vitamin C:	87 mg
Beta carotene:	575 mcg
Calcium:	56 mg
Potassium:	370 mg
Fiber:	3 g

EAT IT! STEAMED OR RAW BROCCOLI IS A KEY VEGETABLE FOR CLEAN-EATING NUTRITION.

BERRIES   5

Berries are tiny packages of power, carrying enormous quantities of disease-fighting antioxidants and a whopping load of fiber. Berries, especially blueberries, should always be on your Clean-Eating superfood list. They are loaded with iron, vitamins A and C, fiber, carotenoids and anthocyanins. Today grocery stores carry them year-round, although there's nothing like wild blues! Eating one cup of berries per day virtually guarantees good health. Try them in salads, cold or hot cereal and in smoothies or just plain, out of the hand.

✳ Calcium

✳ Vitamin C

NUTRIENT VALUE PER ONE-CUP SERVING:

Calories:	30
Vitamin C:	17 mg
Fiber:	2 g
Complex carbohydrates:	57 g
Calcium:	12 mg
Folate:	6 mcg
Carotene:	30 mcg

ENJOY THEM! BEST RIGHT OFF THE BUSH, BERRIES ARE EQUALLY DELICIOUS RAW SITTING ATOP YOUR MORNING OATMEAL AND YOGURT OR AS A SNACK TO APPEASE HUNGER BEFORE BED.

HEARD OF GOJI BERRIES? These are the latest in power-packed berries, straight from the Himalayan Mountains. Containing more antioxidants than any other berry, these are becoming more and more popular with savvy nutritionists and physique enthusiasts. The berries are highly perishable, so the best way to get their goodness is to eat them dried or drink their juice. Ounce for ounce they contain more vitamin C than any other vitamin C-containing food.

BEANS & LEGUMES 6

Beans, sometimes called pulses, are loaded with fiber, vegetable protein and vitamins. Protein from beans is incomplete because it does not contain the amino acid lysine, but adding beans to the diet is a good protein alternative. Beans are a good source of protein, calcium, iron and fiber, which make them perfect for including with Clean-Eating meals. First eaten in ancient times, beans continue to deliver a no-fat, inexpensive and delicious meal today.

STAR NUTRIENTS:

✳ Fiber

✳ Protein

NUTRIENT VALUE PER SIX-OUNCE SERVING:

Calories:	266
Protein:	22 g
Complex carbohydrates:	44 g
Calcium:	100 mg
Iron:	6 mg
Zinc:	3 mg

HARD ON THE TUMMY? SOAK BEANS OVERNIGHT TO ELIMINATE SOME OF THE GAS PROBLEM.

HUMMUS: Instead of fatty dips made with sour cream or mayonnaise, try hummus or bean spreads. Sometimes called white peanut butter, bean dips make a great dip or spread alternative.

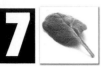

7

SPINACH

In addition to being a Clean-Eating superfood, spinach is my new favorite vegetable. I add it to everything from salads, wraps and soups to omelets and other egg dishes. The deep green color of spinach is a clue that it's loaded with good-for-you nutrients. Spinach contains an abundance of vitamins A, B6, C, E and K along with the minerals iron, calcium, magnesium, manganese and zinc, and the phytochemicals lutein, zeaxanthin, beta-carotene, omega-3 fatty acids, glutathione, alpha lipoic acid, coenzyme Q10, thiamine, riboflavin, folate, vitamin K. The reason for the intense green color of spinach is chlorophyll, which is a potent anti-cancer agent. It is a relatively inexpensive vegetable that can be eaten raw or steamed, for breakfast, lunch or dinner. No wonder Popeye loved his spinach!

✳ STAR NUTRIENTS:

✳ Calcium

✳ Vitamin C

NUTRIENT VALUE PER TWO-CUP SERVING (RAW):

Calories:	25
Potassium:	500 mg
Folate:	150 mcg
Fiber:	2 g
Calcium:	170 mg
Iron:	2 mg
Vitamin C:	26 mg
Vitamin E:	2 mg

EAT SPINACH!

SPINACH LEAVES ARE THE PERFECT FAST-SUPPER FIX. THE LEAVES CAN BE USED IN A SALAD WITH CHOPPED VEGETABLES AND NUTS AND SERVED WITH A GRILLED CHICKEN BREAST OR THEY CAN BE LIGHTLY STEAMED AND SERVED WITH EGG WHITES. THROW THEM INTO A TOMATO SAUCE AND SERVE OVER PASTA.

BODY BUILDING: Women should eat plenty of spinach since it is low in calories and high in fiber and vitamins, but most importantly it contains plenty of calcium, important for bone health.

WALNUTS

8

One of the world's oldest foods, walnuts were once considered a symbol of fertility and were always included in the marriage beds of newlyweds in ancient Rome. Walnuts have the highest overall antioxidant activity of all nuts. The delicious nut contains melatonin, ellagic acid, gamma tocopherol, carotenoids and polyphenols. It is also one of the few nuts that contain plenty of omega-3 fatty acids, important for combating inflammation and obesity. Rather than put weight on, which most people think any nuts will do, walnuts help to fill you up and satisfy you as a result of their high fiber, fat and protein content. Be sure to add nuts to your Clean-Eating regimen.

✳ STAR NUTRIENTS:

✳ Omega-3 fatty acids

✳ Vitamin E

NUTRIENT VALUE PER 100 GRAMS OR 3.5 OUNCES:

Calories:	688
Protein:	15 g
Fat:	69 g
Calcium:	94 mg
Vitamin E:	4 mg
Iron:	3 mg
Zinc:	3 mg

STORAGE: Walnuts and other nuts are oily and can go rancid quickly if improperly stored. Always store nuts in a cool, dry place in an airtight container. I buy them whole and keep them in the refrigerator.

EAT THEM: WALNUTS ARE A VERSATILE FOOD. THEY CAN BE USED FOR COOKING, BAKING AND JUST PLAIN EATING.

BISON – THE OTHER RED MEAT

This rich red protein source is also known as buffalo. Bison offers a pleasant taste surprise. It's tender like beef but sweeter and richer in flavor. It is not at all gamey, since it is not raised like conventional beef cattle with hormone- and antibiotic-laced feed. Bison is an excellent protein source. Bison can be eaten in place of red meat without the worry of added fat or cholesterol. The meat can be ground for use in burgers and stews. Nutritionists are beginning to recommend bison over beef for its superior nutrition profile. I like to include it in my Clean-Eating menu because it is a low-fat red-meat alternative. Most other red meats are too fatty.

✳ STAR NUTRIENTS:

✳ Protein

✳ Calcium

NUTRITIONAL VALUE PER FOUR-OUNCE SERVING:

Calories:	123
Protein:	24 g
Fat:	2.4 g
Saturated fat:	0.8 g
Cholesterol:	75 mg
Calcium:	9 mg

HEART HEALTHY! The American Heart Association recommends eating bison meat because of its nutritional profile and low-fat, low-cholesterol status.

CONJUGATED LINOLEIC ACID: Bison meat is one of the few meats high in CLA, which has been found useful in promoting weight loss.

HALF THE CALORIES: BISON MEAT HAS HALF THE CALORIES OF PORK OR CHICKEN.

www.thebuffaloshop.com
www.montanabison.org

. . . .

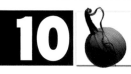

10 PUMPKIN

First Nations peoples on the continent of North America cultivated and thus survived on the dense, orange flesh of pumpkins. Pumpkin flesh is usually reserved for Thanksgiving and Christmas, and of course the happy gourd is central to the celebration of Halloween, yet pumpkins and brightly colored sweet potatoes can be eaten sweet or savory year-round. They are an inexpensive food, dense with nutrients and fiber. The bright orange flesh of pumpkins indicates that they are loaded with the powerful antioxidant beta-carotene. In fact, one cup of boiled pumpkin provides 310 percent of the recommended daily allowance of vitamin A. I feel good just looking at a pumpkin, but it's far better to eat this Clean-Eating superfood than simply look at it.

✳ STAR NUTRIENTS:

✳ Carotenoids, especially beta carotene

✳ Fiber

NUTRIENT VALUE PER ONE-CUP SERVING:

Calories:	49
Carbohydrates:	12 g
Alpha carotene:	28 mcg
Beta carotene:	900 mcg
Fiber:	3 g
Vitamin C:	28 mg
Vitamin E:	2 mg

DID YOU KNOW? PUMPKINS ARE 90 PERCENT WATER.

SEEDS: Pumpkin seeds are also a nutritional superstar. They are full of zinc and essential fatty acids.

PUMPKIN-SEED VIAGRA? Pumpkin seeds contain loads of zinc, which help stimulate the libido! They are a lot cheaper than Viagra, too.
www.pumpkinnook.com
www.punkinranch.com

. . . .

SOY   **11**

The soybean is actually a legume, but it stands in a class of its own because it contains so many nutrients. Initially considered a food for Asians and health nuts only, soy is becoming more mainstream since it's hard to argue with its nutritional profile. Soy foods seem to have a positive effect on several conditions, including heart disease and menopause. Soybean-based products contain all of the essential amino acids. This is rare for a plant. Soybeans are an excellent source of B vitamins, potassium, zinc and other minerals, as well as soluble fiber and omega-3 fatty acids. Soy is an inexpensive complete source of protein and should appear on your Clean-Eating menu several times per week.

✳ STAR NUTRIENTS:

✳ Protein

✳ Phytoestrogens

✳ Omega-3 fatty acids

NUTRIENT VALUE PER FOUR-OUNCE SERVING:

Calories:	370
Protein:	36 g
Calcium:	240 mg
Iron:	10 mg
Fiber:	16 g
Zinc:	4 mg

SOY, THE VERSATILE PROTEIN: Soy protein is made from soy-bean curd. It readily takes on the flavors of other foods it is cooked with, so it can taste the way you like it.

EAT MORE SOY!
INCORPORATE SOY-BASED PRODUCTS INTO YOUR DIET BY ADDING SOY PROTEIN TO A SMOOTHIE, USING FIRM TOFU IN STIR-FRIES AND DRINKING SOY BEVERAGES. YOU CAN ALSO LOOK FOR SOY-BASED CEREALS, BREAD AND YOGURT.

www.talksoy.com
www.soynutrition.com

OATMEAL   12

A bowl brimming with hot oatmeal or one of its whole-grain cousins is one of the best ways to start your day. Sugary cereals like Froot Loops or Cinnamon Toast Crunch don't come within a mile of the nutritional power of oats. Slow-burning complex carbohydrates in oatmeal prolong the feeling of fullness and prevent blood sugar from rising wildly. These are important factors when changing nutrition habits. You want to feel full longer. The soluble fiber in oatmeal fills you while lowering blood cholesterol. Oatmeal also contains plant protein, essential for building muscle. Oatmeal is one of the few foods rich in silicon, a mineral responsible for building beautiful skin, hair, bones and teeth. Oats also contain phosphorus, essential for brain and nerve growth during youth. This is dependable Clean-Eating food at its best.

✳ STAR NUTRIENTS:

✳ Soluble fiber

✳ Protein

✳ Complex carbohydrates

✳ Silicon

NUTRIENT VALUE PER ONE-CUP SERVING (COOKED):	
Calories:	149
Fiber:	7 g
Protein:	6 g
Carbohydrates:	25 g
Iron:	1 g

REV UP YOUR OATMEAL: Oatmeal on its own is a superior food but when you add one tablespoon each of ground flaxseed, bee pollen and wheat germ you really rev up the its nutritional profile. Add fresh berries and you've increased your nutrition substantially.

OATMEAL MAKES HEALTH HISTORY: IN 1997 OATMEAL MADE HISTORY WHEN THE FDA ALLOWED IT TO BE THE FIRST FOOD TO BE LABELED "HEART HEALTHY." OATS HAVE BEEN SCIENTIFICALLY PROVEN TO LOWER BLOOD CHOLESTEROL IF EATEN REGULARLY.

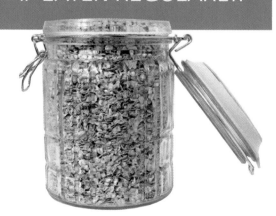

YOU'RE DESTROYING YOUR NUTRIENTS!

There are a number of things you are doing to destroy any nutrients you are getting. *Some examples are:*

- Overeating
- Eating standing up
- Rush-eating
- Not chewing adequately or properly
- Eating after 6:00 pm and late into the night
- Consuming too much caffeine, alcohol, nicotine, marijuana, drugs
- Consuming too much sugar, fake or otherwise, flour, and refined and over-processed foods
- Consuming too many chemicals lurking in food and water
- Over-dependence on antibiotics and man-made drugs
- Treating symptoms of disease instead of the cause

NUTRITION PRIORITIES
THE PLAN FOR GETTING YOU ON TRACK

1 Eliminate poor foods

2 Replace poor-quality foods with high-quality, Clean-Eating foods

3 Supplement with superfoods and vitamins

4 Reduce overindulgence

TOP SUPPLEMENTS

I have included a section on supplements in this book not to push supplementation, but to handle this controversial subject head on. Every second question I field from readers seems to be about whether or not to supplement their nutrition or to take supplements in any form. Let's take a step back and consider that supplements are a good thing if you take the definition literally – they are simply products or foods we take in addition to our daily food to improve our health. Vitamins qualify as a supplement. So do bee pollen, wheat germ, flaxseed, EFAs (essential fatty acids), wheat grass, chlorophyll and a host of others. They are "nice-to-have" additions in our daily diet.

Where the water gets muddy is with "supplements" that may or may not help you lose weight, and there are an abundance of these since nearly two-thirds of us claim to be on a diet at any given time. Some of these products can in fact assist you (albeit fractionally) and others do nothing at all. I do not recommend taking any supplements of this nature if you feel your nutrition is acceptable. If you wish to push the envelope a little and bump up your fat burning then consider some of these, but again not all, and not because I said so.

Do your own research and always be skeptical, very skeptical of what a company is trying to encourage you to consume. If you are considering taking hoodia, for example, then make sure that the first ingredient on the label is indeed hoodia and that it is present in good concentration. Otherwise you might as well toss your hard earned dollars into the Mississippi River.

As with anything in life, balance is the way to approach supplementation. Whenever I can get my nutrients from food, I do. But I have always been the type of person who likes to eat my food rather than take it in pill form.

CO-ENZYME Q10

Coenzyme Q10 is a powerful antioxidant developed in Japan after the dropping of the Hiroshima bomb. Its main functions are as a free-radical scavenger and to provide energy for the body's cell growth and maintenance. Every cell in the body already contains this fat-soluble substance. It helped the people of Japan fight the devastating effects of the bomb and it can certainly help you. One remarkable aspect of CoQ10 is its ability to drive metabolic reactions in the body more efficiently. Mitochondria contain the greatest amount of Coenzyme Q10. Our bodies produce CoQ10 but as we age levels of this critical antioxidant drop. This reduction is made worse by poor nutrition.

Coenzyme Q10 also stimulates the immune system and protects the heart from damage caused by chemotherapy treatments. Lately CoQ10 has been used to treat gum disease and Raynaud's syndrome. The recommended daily dosage is 100 to 200 mg, but you would have to eat the equivalent of 3 1/2 pounds of sardines, 6 pounds of beef or 8 pounds of peanuts to get 100 milligrams of CoQ10. That is an improbable task for anyone. Luckily, CoQ10 is available as a potent man-made supplement.

DOSAGE: The recommended daily dosage is 100 to 200 mg or more depending on your condition.

DID YOU KNOW? Peter D. Mitchell, Ph.D., of the University of Edinburgh, won the Nobel Prize for chemistry in 1978 for figuring out how CoQ10 produces energy at the cellular level.

Green Coenzyme Q10 is also known as ubiquinone.

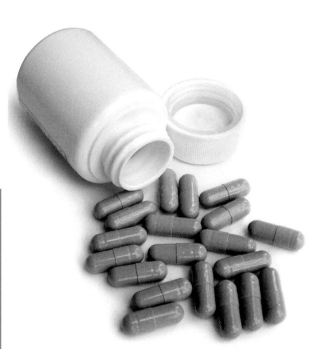

CREATINE

Much has been made of illicit muscle-building steroids in the news lately with every professional athlete from those who play baseball to cyclists, football players and sprinters getting involved and getting into trouble. Steroids are illegal and destructive to health over the long term. However, creatine is legitimately known as a supplement that can safely help the body build muscle. Remember, the more lean muscle you have the higher your metabolic rate. Creatine exists naturally in human muscle but to a higher degree in skeletal muscle. It assists the body by increasing the amount of energy available in muscle. Meat and fish are the richest sources of naturally occurring creatine. The best of these include raw tuna, sushi or sashimi. Raw is best because heating creatine degrades it. Not everyone enjoys raw fish, so supplementation is an option. Creatine plays a critical role in lowering blood levels of the dangerous agent homocysteine. Homocysteine has been linked to diseases including Alzheimers, Parkinson's, stroke and vascular disease. Creatine is also capable of lowering plasma cholesterol.

HOW IS IT SOLD? Synthetic creatine is commonly used to enhance athletic performance. It is sold as citrate, phosphate or monohydrate salts.

HOW MUCH? The recommended dosage ranges from 2 to 20 grams. This is a supplement where it's not best to consume more. Check with your doctor first if you have concerns or questions, although a prescription is not required.

QUALITY: Manufacturers like to add fillers, so be sure to check the label before you make your creatine purchase. Check for added refined or fake sugar.

CONJUGATED LINOLEIC ACID/CLA

Conjugated linoleic acid, or CLA, is a supplement used to promote fat loss and the growth of lean muscle tissue. It is highly effective in assisting with weight loss and seems capable of changing your body composition. If you are struggling to lose stubborn fat deposits around your midsection, CLA seems to be effective at doing just that. If you've already lost weight and want to keep the weight off, studies indicate it can help by increasing your basal metabolic rate.

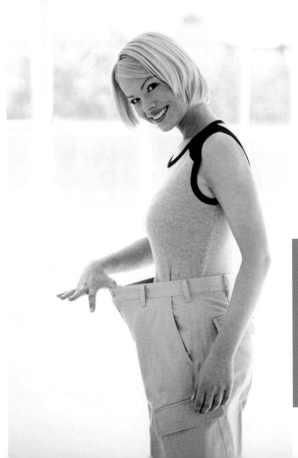

The action of CLA is that it prevents lipogenesis, or the storage of fat in adipose tissue, after a meal. CLA is a structured lipid or essential fatty acid occurring naturally in beef, ground turkey, lamb, cheese and milk. We have become suspicious of fats as they have earned a negative reputation. While it is true that certain fats are not beneficial, the body does require EFAs for health and to utilize nutrients properly.

To get the optimal amount of CLA you would have to consume enormous quantities of these foods. By doing so you would end up eating too many calories which is counteractive for weight loss. Instead you can supplement. CLA also acts as an antioxidant and enhances the immune system.

DOSAGE: 1-3 g or 1000-3000 mg

TRANS FAT: CLA is actually a trans fat, but in this case a beneficial one.

BEE POLLEN

I love bee pollen and add one tablespoon to my cereal along with ground flaxseed and wheat germ every morning. It readily dissolves in hot or cold liquids. Bee pollen is valued for its complete array of proteins, vitamins, minerals and enzymes. Bee pollen supports every bodily system, with emphasis on the nervous and reproductive systems. Scientists suggest bee pollen is a complete food. The protein in bee pollen is easily digestible and readily accessible for use in the body. The tiny golden orbs contain

Eat some half an hour before meals on an empty stomach to help you fight hunger pains.

powerful antioxidants, which have been proven to reduce the threat of free-radical damage from everyday toxins.

Bee pollen is known for its high rutin levels. Rutin is a quercetin found in many plants, especially buckwheat, green tea and apple skins. Rutin strengthens capillaries and therefore improves cardiovascular endurance. Since pollen is so easily digested and absorbed on an empty stomach it can lessen hunger between meals. Eat one teaspoon half an hour before meals on an empty stomach to help you fight hunger pains. It is delicious eaten as a snack if you can't hold out until your next meal.

Bee pollen contains an alphabet soup of nutrients, including the B vitamins: B1, B2, B3, B5, B6 and B12; vitamins A, C and E, carotenoids, folic acid and rutin; minerals, including magnesium, calcium, copper, iron, silica, phosphorus, sulfur, chlorine and manganese. It contains a full range of amino acids and is a more concentrated source of protein than any other food. On top of all of that it contains necessary digestive enzymes, fatty acids and a full range of phytonutrients. Everyone can benefit from taking at least one teaspoon of bee pollen per day.

If you are worried about allergies, especially pollen allergies, use bee pollen cautiously at the beginning. Introduce your body to it by taking a few grains at a time for a few days. If there is no allergic reaction you'll be fine to increase the amount to one tea-spoon per day. Otherwise stop taking it.

WEBSITES OFFERING BEE POLLEN:
www.philoxia.com
www.honeygardens.com

HOLY BASIL OR TULSI

Known as "tulsi" or the "the incomparable one" in Ayurvedic medicine, the herb tulsi has been revered for its health-promoting and medicinal qualities for thousands of years in India. Tulsi contains hundreds of beneficial phytochemicals working in synergy. Holy basil is highly effective at regulating the body's response to stress, primarily the cortisol response. It is called an adaptogen, or an agent that improves the fighting capacity of the body against stress. In the 21st century we are under a constant barrage of stress. As a result, stress hormones pour into our system all day long; our bodies never have a chance to rest. Cortisol is one of these stress hormones. Its job is to increase blood sugar levels so there is plenty of fuel available for the body in a fight-or-flight situation. It also maintains blood pressure during times of stress. Blood sugar acts as a fuel source, but the overstressed lives we lead add up to excessive cortisol and therefore excessive blood sugar. Add to that the toxins we absorb from pollution, cigarettes, coffee, alcohol and more and we are in trouble. Tulsi regulates cortisol during situations of stress, helping to normalize blood-sugar levels. (Consistently high glucose levels increase the risk of developing diabetes and overweight since excess sugar is stored as fat.) Tulsi also helps to relieve anxiety and depression.

DRINK IT! Even one cup of tulsi tea per day is benefi-cial. Drinking more will maximize your health.

ORGANIC BRANDS: Look for organic brands con-taining pure and natural ingredients. The taste is pleasant and sweet.

www.organicindia.com

HOODIA

Hoodia is a succulent, or fruit of the cactus plant, used by the San Bushmen of the Kalahari Desert. They used this cucumber-like fruit to quench thirst and to ward off hunger. It served them well in their harsh environment and with their nomadic lifestyle. Scientists have now discovered that Hoodia gordonii causes weight loss in animals. Today it is used as an appetite suppressant.

In the July 2005 issue of *Oprah*, the new genera-tion of diet pills was reviewed, Hoodia among them.

Supplement manufacturers excitedly jumped on the bandwagon. It seemed this could finally be the magic weight-loss pill everyone was looking for. There must be something quite different in the actual plant than in the supplement, though. As Oprah's writer reports, "So far however, there's little proof that the supplements are even mildly effective: Most contain only small, probably insignificant levels of Hoodia extract and caffeine is likely the active ingredient in many of them." No one has been able to determine how Hoodia works.

DOSAGE: Most companies recommend a dosage of 400 mg to 700 mg.

BUYER BEWARE! Because Hoodia shows so much promise, many supplement manufacturers ran with the idea, flooding the market with product. Be careful what you buy. There are loads of cheap imitations that do not produce results. Choose a reputable source where the product is 100 percent Hoodia. Expect to pay for real Hoodia, it is expensive. The best

Hoodia comes from South Africa, where the plant originated. Only the core and stems contain the effective Hoodia ingredients.

HGH – HUMAN GROWTH HORMONE

The body produces its own growth hormone, most of it while you are in a deep sleep, and mainly while you are in your youth. According to **Oz Garcia**, author of *Look and Feel Fabulous Forever,* "a deficiency of hGH impacts on, well … everything, especially by increasing the volume of fat and abdominal obesity we store, and by reducing muscle mass and strength. A drop in your natural production of hGH is a direct pathway to flab."

The key seems to be getting enough sleep, but it is more than that. Your sleep must be of a good quality. If you are up all night heading for the bathroom or the refrigerator you aren't sleeping well. The quality of your sleep is also compromised when you snore or have sleep apnea. Don't underestimate sleep as an ideal way to both control weight and produce plenty of hGH.

There are non-prescription products available, called pro hGH. These products stimulate the production of natural hGH. Garcia further states, "In your twenties you may 'release' GH about 12 times a day during a 24-hour period. After the age of 30, the number and intensity of 'releases' drop 14 percent for every decade you're alive." Among its benefits, pro hGH products improve muscle strength and size, reduce fat and increase the ability to exercise.

As baby boomers get older they seek to fight both aging and weight gain. Human growth hormone is fast becoming a factor in both cases because it increases our ability to burn fat faster. Somehow hGH causes fat cells in adipose tissue to shrink so they are less able to hold fat.

AVAILABILITY: Actual hGH is available only by prescription and as an injectable. The cost is prohibitive at US $600 per injection and you would need to inject yourself every day. Injected hGH is also implicated in an increased risk of prostate cancer in men. If you do choose to take hGH you must see a doctor during the course of your therapy.

NATURAL HGH STIMULATION: The three most effective ways to stimulate your own hGH production are to sleep well, eat enough protein, and exercise.

WHEY PROTEIN

Most of us, especially women, do not consume enough high-quality protein. What meat we do consume is often loaded with chemicals, hormones and unnecessary fat. In order to keep muscle tissue nourished, your body requires protein, especially if you are active and train with weights. Protein needs must be met to keep the body strong and to prevent muscle from

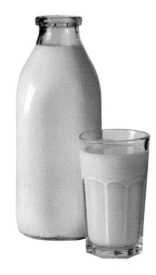

catabolizing itself. In other words, if you don't consume enough protein, your body consumes its own muscle in order to meet its protein requirements.

According to **Dr. Deborah Chud**, author of *The Gourmet Prescription*, "Protein, fat and fiber act as brakes on the insulin production machine because they slow the digestion of food. The slower our food is digested, the more gradually our blood- sugar levels rise and the slower the production of insulin." An essential element of Clean Eating, protein consumed at every meal, supports this mechanism. It is essential and smart to include protein with every meal, as Clean Eating advocates. Not only does protein contain all 22 amino acids necessary for building and repairing healthy tissue, it contains vitamins, minerals, fatty acids and natural detoxifying agents.

"Whey is just the powder left after the cream has been skimmed off and the milk put through a drying process. It has virtually no fat but all the nutritional goodness of milk. Milk is the exclusive food used by all mammals to grow healthy," states Robert Kennedy, publisher of *Oxygen* magazine. "This supplement is used more than any other by all those seeking to trim and define their physique." Whey powders contain an array of micronutrients, antioxidants and immunoglobulins that help sustain overall health. Look for whey powders low in carbohydrates and fats. Check the nutrition label for unnecessary sugars, both refined and fake.

DOSAGE: Protein should be consumed every three hours. Protein powder can be added to hot cereal, shakes, smoothies and yogurt.

CAN'T DO WHEY? Look for other all-natural protein powders, such as hemp or soy.

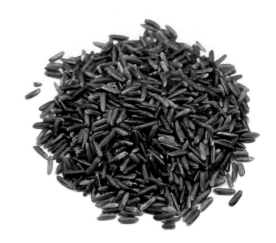

GAMMA-ORYZANOL AND BROWN RICE

There is no good reason to eat white rice if you can eat brown. The nutritional value of brown rice is far superior. There are so many interesting varieties that you'll never get bored, and the taste is superb. Beyond its culinary attributes, unrefined brown rice possesses the ability to reduce blood-sugar levels. This is an important consideration in the fight against overweight and obesity. I recommend eating brown rice in the Clean-Eating plan.

The bran that coats each grain of brown rice "is thought to be one of the most nutrient-dense substances ever studied," states the author of *Healing With Whole Foods*, **Paul Pitchford**. "It embodies over 70 antioxidants that can protect against cellular damage and preserve youthfulness." Rice bran contains the rare form of vitamin E known as tocotrienol, which assists the body in lowering fat and cholesterol. Polysaccharides, also found in rice bran, are complex carbs ideally suited for controlling high blood sugar, the implicating factor in diabetes and obesity.

Gamma-oryzanol is a potent antioxidant, and rice bran is a good source. This compound has the ability to strengthen muscles. Brown rice bran also contains loads of CoQ10, another super supplement already discussed in this chapter.

EXCHANGE: Instead of buying white rice next time you are at the grocery store, exchange it for brown rice. There are so many wonderful kinds available. You and your family deserve to have this valuable food on your dinner table.

DOSAGE: Gamma-oryzanol can be purchased as a supplemental oil. Take one teaspoon per day.

OMEGA-3 FATTY ACIDS

There are three essential fatty acids required for overall good health. Omega-3 in particular has been proven to regulate appetite and to accelerate fat burning. That's a very good thing when you are trying to lose weight. I often think people would be healthier if omegas-3, 6 and 9 did not have the word "fat" attached to them. Everyone shuns fat but the consumption of these fatty acids is beneficial. Omega-3 is found in good supply in fish and flaxseed. It contains ALA, or alpha-linolenic acid, which reduces fat storage – obviously helpful in managing overweight and obesity.

Omega-3 fats are the most valuable players on the fat team. The best sources are oily, cold-water fish, including mackerel, salmon, herring and sardines. Another way of getting omega-3 in your diet is through plant products. The best sources include flaxseed, hempseed, pumpkin seed and rapeseed. Dark green leafy vegetables like kale, collard greens, purslane and parsley are also good sources because they contain ALA in their chloroplasts.

FISH CONSUMPTION: Seven to ten ounces of fish per week.

DOSAGE OF FLAX PRODUCTS: Work your way up to four tablespoons of ground flaxseed with meals each day.

LEAFY GREENS: Eat them every day!

MACA

Maca is a powerful adaptogenic agent derived from a nutritious root vegetable originally grown in the harsh climate of the Andes Mountains. Peruvian peoples have depended on this wrinkled root as a valuable source of nutrition for thousands of years. It can withstand both freezing winds and intense sunlight in these remote places. It is grown without

pesticides or chemicals. Maca's rich nutritional content is one of the reasons it is so valuable, especially for those with weakened immune systems. It contains 31 trace minerals, and this is particularly important today in view of the highly processed foods we normally consume. (Processed foods rob the body of minerals.)

Athletes use maca to increase energy, stamina and endurance. It is used as a safe alternative to anabolic steroids because the root is rich in sterols, natural plant hormone-like substances. Recently a major US baseball team used maca as part of their nutrition program after the head coach discovered his energy was enhanced when he consumed it. The nutrients in maca are readily digestible and therefore immediately accessible to the body. Results are felt soon after taking it. Since it is a food it is entirely safe to take and is of immense health benefit.

DOSAGE: Available over the counter as a powder, pill or tea. Take 1500 to 3000 mg per day.

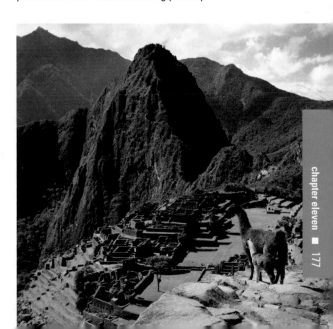

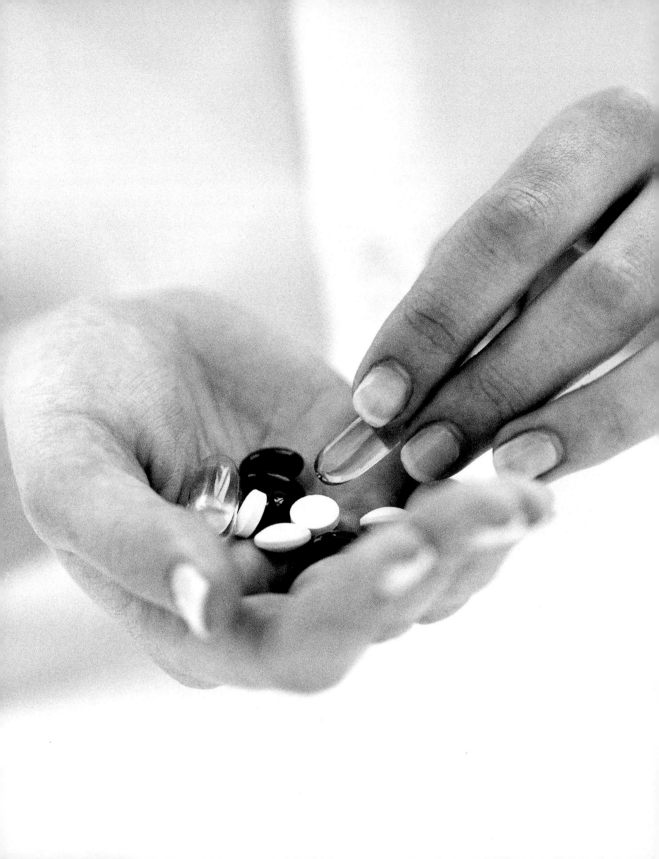

FLAXSEED

I already mentioned a few benefits of flaxseed in the omega-3 section. I have to admit that since it is indeed a food I greatly debated whether to put it under the heading of superfoods or supplements.

If I had to choose only one supplement it would be flaxseed. You already know about its omega-3 content, but it has many other health benefits. Flaxseed has 27 identifiable cancer-preventative compounds. Many experts recommend it for breast and prostate cancer prevention. It has also been shown to aid in the regulation of blood sugar, and to lower LDL (bad) cholesterol and blood pressure.

If all of this isn't enough, you should know that people who consume it daily show an increased metabolic rate and are leaner on average than those who do not. It also does wonders for your skin and hair.

Have troubles with constipation? (Hey, this stuff is important!) A daily dose of flaxseed cures that quickly! Here's a funny story: I found out that a friend of mine had been suffering from constipation for many years. I told her to try flaxseed, starting with only a ¼ tablespoon a day and eventually working up to 2 to 4 tablespoons (I take four). This woman, a teacher, phoned me later to tell me she had a very embarrassing day in class because she kept running to the bathroom. It turned out she thought I told her to take a ¼ cup of flaxseed! Well, we straightened that mess out (no pun intended) and she is now as regular as the best of us. And you

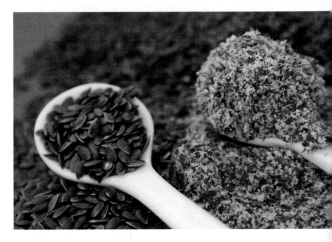

know what else happened? She lost 10 pounds! Just like that.

On top of all of this, I have heard reports that flaxseed helps with menopausal symptoms, enhances your immune system, alleviates inflammatory conditions and even helps with ADD. Phew! That's a long list of benefits from one little seed!

DOSAGE: Start with one teaspoon a day and gradually work your way up to four tablespoons per day. Dr. Bob Arnott recommends four tablespoons (¼ cup) daily to help prevent breast cancer.

NOTE: Make sure to grind your flaxseed before consumption. If you eat the seeds whole they will simply pass right through your system, and you will not receive the benefits. I prefer grinding the seeds myself in a coffee grinder because pre-ground seeds will have lost some of their nutritional value and they are more likely to be rancid. To keep your seeds fresher longer store them in a cool, dark place. I store mine in the refrigerator.

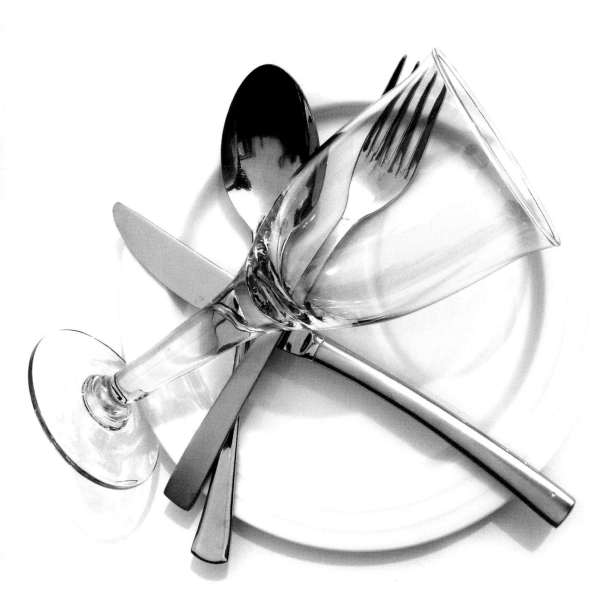

CHAPTER TWELVE

EAT-CLEAN
MENUS

COOLER 1 MEAL PLAN

	MORNING START	MIDMORNING BOOSTER	LUNCHTIME REFUEL
DAY 1	Oatmeal with flaxseed, wheat germ and bee pollen; egg whites; black coffee, distilled water or green tea	Grilled chicken breast; ½ sweet potato; distilled water	Water-packed tuna served with lettuce and cucumbers and squeeze of fresh lemon juice; 1 apple; distilled water
DAY 2	Quinoa with flaxseed, wheat germ and bee pollen; egg whites; black coffee, distilled water or green tea	Water-packed tuna with sliced cucumbers and radishes; distilled water	Turkey breast (not deli meat) with ½ sweet potato and spinach; distilled water
DAY 3	Cream of Wheat with flaxseed, wheat germ and bee pollen; egg whites; black coffee, distilled water or green tea	Grilled chicken breast with sliced celery; distilled water	Water-packed tuna with lettuce and tomato with a squeeze of fresh lemon juice; distilled water
DAY 4	Brown rice with flaxseed, wheat germ and bee pollen; egg whites; black coffee, distilled water or green tea	Water-packed tuna; sliced cucumbers; distilled water	Grilled chicken breast with ½ sweet potato wilted spinach with lemon; distilled water
DAY 5	Oatmeal with flaxseed, wheat germ and bee pollen; egg whites; black coffee, distilled water or green tea	Chicken breast with green beans; distilled water	Turkey with ½ sweet potato served with lettuce and tomatoes with a squeeze of fresh lemon juice; distilled water
DAY 6	Quinoa with flaxseed, wheat germ and bee pollen; egg whites; black coffee, distilled water or green tea	Lean ground turkey with chopped tomato and zucchini; distilled water	Tuna loin with ½ sweet potato; apple; distilled water
DAY 7	Cream of Wheat with flaxseed, wheat germ and bee pollen; egg whites; black coffee, distilled water or green tea	Hardboiled egg whites with sliced cucumbers and tomato; distilled water	Chicken breast; ½ sweet potato; green beans; distilled water

Here are some Eat-Clean menus and grocery lists to show you how you might choose to eat throughout the week. They are simply suggested guidelines. Adjust portion sizes accordingly (refer to page 39). "Morning Start" should be consumed whenever you wake up. Each subsequent meal is eaten 2 ½ to 3 hours thereafter. The "Before Bed" meal should be eaten only if you are hungry and if you are not following the Cooler 1 meal plan.

MIDAFTER-NOON MUNCH	DINNER DELIGHT
Scrambled egg whites served with tomatoes; distilled water	Lean turkey breast served with green beans and ½ sweet potato; distilled water
Egg-white omelet with tomatoes; 1 apple; distilled water	Chicken with ½ sweet potato and green beans; distilled water
Turkey breast; ½ sweet potato; distilled water	Tilapia with ½ sweet potato and mixed greens; distilled water
Hardboiled egg whites sliced over a bed of greens with chopped celery and a squeeze of lemon juice; distilled water	Turkey breast with ½ sweet potato and steamed zucchini; distilled water
Scrambled egg whites with spinach and onion; distilled water	Tuna loin; ½ sweet potato; apple; distilled water
Hardboiled egg whites with asparagus; distilled water	Grilled chicken; ½ sweet potato; green beans; distilled water
Chopped celery, apple and water-packed tuna; distilled water	Bison with ½ sweet potato and asparagus; distilled water

COOLER 1 GROCERY LIST*

PRODUCE

- ❑ Tomatoes
- ❑ Zucchini
- ❑ Cucumber
- ❑ Celery
- ❑ Sweet potatoes
- ❑ Green beans
- ❑ Asparagus
- ❑ Apples
- ❑ Spinach
- ❑ Radishes
- ❑ Lettuce
- ❑ Lemons

DAIRY

- ❑ Egg whites

GRAINS

- ❑ Oatmeal
- ❑ Cream of Wheat
- ❑ Quinoa
- ❑ Brown rice

BUTCHER

- ❑ Lean ground turkey
- ❑ Lean turkey breast
- ❑ Boneless, skinless chicken breast
- ❑ Bison tenderloin
- ❑ Water-packed tuna
- ❑ Tuna loin
- ❑ Tilapia

NUTS AND SEEDS

- ❑ Flaxseed

MISCELLANEOUS

- ❑ Distilled water
- ❑ Wheat germ
- ❑ Bee pollen
- ❑ Coffee
- ❑ Green tea

*Grocery lists for the other meal plans begin on page 190.

FAMILY MEAL PLAN

NOTE: The family meal plan follows cooler 2.

	MORNING START	MIDMORNING BOOSTER	LUNCHTIME REFUEL
DAY 1	Sweet Inca Porridge (p. 246); water and black coffee or green tea	Fat-free cottage cheese; apple; water	Mixed greens; sliced tomatoes; grilled chicken; a squeeze of lemon; piece of Ezekiel toast; water
DAY 2	Fat-free yogurt with raspberries, flax seed, bee pollen, wheat germ and a scoop of vanilla protein powder; Ezekiel toast; water and black coffee or green tea	Pear; handful of unsalted almonds; water	Whole-grain wrap spread with yogurt cheese and topped with salsa, alfalfa sprouts and hardboiled egg whites; water
DAY 3	Whole-grain cereal with skim milk, flaxseed, wheat germ, bee pollen, sliced banana, scrambled egg whites; water and black coffee or green tea	Celery stalks, rinsed, spread with nut butter and topped with raisins; water	Ezekiel bread spread with hummus; leftover sliced Parchment-Baked Chicken placed on top with spinach and onions; water
DAY 4	Small whole-grain wrap with scrambled egg whites; topped with tomatoes and mushrooms; water and black coffee or green tea	Almond butter on rice cakes; apple; water	Leftover turkey breast on baby spinach salad with sprouts and other mixed greens, spritzed with lemon juice; water
DAY 5	Oatmeal pancakes topped with applesauce and sliced strawberries; scrambled egg whites; water and black coffee or green tea	1 Clean protein bar; water	Thai Beef Salad (pg. 228); water
DAY 6	Potato, Rocket and Tomato Frittata (p. 204); water and black coffee or green tea	Smoothie made with berries, vanilla protein powder and rice milk; water	Quinoa, tomatoes, and cucumber with tofu, balsamic vinaigrette and olive oil; water
DAY 7	Oatmeal with berries, wheat germ, bee pollen, flaxseed; hardboiled egg whites; water and black coffee or green tea	1 Tbsp almond butter spread on brown-rice cakes; apple; water	Leek and Potato Soup (p. 216); hummus spread on Salba crackers; water

MIDAFTER-NOON MUNCH	DINNER DELIGHT	BEFORE BED IF HUNGRY
Whole-grain wrap spread with nut butter and topped with sliced banana; water	Steamed sea bass; Summertime Risotto (p. 227), asparagus and red pepper; water	Leftover Sweet Inca Porridge; water or herbal tea
Sliced cucumbers, carrots, and red pepper, with hummus and Salba crackers; water	Parchment-Baked Chicken with Arugula, Sage and Rosemary (p. 212); quinoa; steamed broccoli; water	Smoothie made with protein powder, banana, blueberries, vanilla, nonfat yogurt and dash of agave nectar; water
Hardboiled egg whites and green peppers mixed with chick peas and salsa; water	Roasted turkey breast; roasted sweet potato, rutabaga, and carrots; water	Cooked oatmeal with unsweetened applesauce and vanilla protein powder; water or herbal tea
Hummus with sliced carrots, cucumbers and cherry tomatoes; water	Chicken and White Bean Soup (p. 207) paired with Ezekiel toast; water	Nonfat plain yogurt with mango and vanilla; water or herbal tea
Fat-free cottage cheese with kiwi slices; water	Grilled salmon fillets; brown rice; Stir-Fried Bok Choy; water	Fat-free yogurt with sliced banana; water or herbal tea
Hummus with crudités; water	Grilled Breast of Chicken Marsala with Grilled Carrots (p.203); water	2 cups unbuttered, air popped popcorn; 1 handful unsalted nuts; water or herbal tea
Clean protein bar; water	Whole-grain pasta noodles with Turkey Meatballs (p. 232), asparagus, spinach and mushrooms; water	Quinoa Fun Dessert (p. 216); water or herbal tea

VEGAN MEAL PLAN

		MORNING START	MIDMORNING BOOSTER	LUNCHTIME REFUEL
DAY 1		Sweet Inca Porridge (p. 246); water, black coffee, or green tea	Pear; handful raw almonds; water	Grilled and diced tofu; mixed greens with a squeeze of lemon juice; brown rice; water
DAY 2		Whole-grain wrap spread with soy yogurt cheese and topped with salsa, alfalfa sprouts and sliced tofu; water	Hummus; carrot, cucumber and red pepper slices; water	Black beans stir-fried with mushrooms, green onions and tomatoes; brown rice; water, black coffee, or green tea
DAY 3		Oatmeal with hemp milk, flaxseed, wheat germ, bee pollen, and berries; water, black coffee, or green tea	Brown rice cakes spread with nut butter; water	Leftover Soybean Dinner Loaf on a whole-wheat wrap with alfalfa sprouts, hummus, and sliced cucumbers; water
DAY 4		Smoothie with cooked oatmeal, applesauce, cinnamon, nutmeg, and 1 scoop of hemp protein powder; water, black coffee, or green tea	Whole-grain bread spread with nut butter and topped with fresh sliced strawberries; water	Stellar Legume Soup (p. 238)**; water
DAY 5		Cinnamon-raisin Ezekiel toast topped with all-natural peanut butter and sliced apple; water, black coffee, or green tea	Smoothie: vanilla soy protein powder, rice milk, cubed mango, raspberries, flaxseed, wheat germ, nonfat soy yogurt; water	Mixed greens paired with chickpeas, black beans, tomatoes, celery, carrots, and cucumbers; squeeze of lemon juice; 1 piece of whole-grain toast; water
DAY 6		Oatmeal with soy vanilla protein powder, flaxseed, bee pollen, raspberries, blueberries and banana; water, black coffee, or green tea	Handful of almonds with fat-free soy yogurt and 1 apple; water	1 warm whole-wheat wrap filled with black beans, edamame, red and green peppers, onions, tomatoes and alfalfa sprouts; water
DAY 7		Dried (Clean) muesli with hemp milk; water, black coffee, or green tea	Clean protein bar; water	Leek and Potato Soup (p. 216)** with hummus spread on Salba crackers; water

* replace chicken broth with vegetable broth; replace turkey breast with diced extra firm tofu
** replace chicken broth with vegetable broth; water
*** replace yogurt with unsweetened soy yogurt

MIDAFTER-NOON MUNCH	DINNER DELIGHT	BEFORE BED IF HUNGRY
Textured vegetable protein cooked with onions and garlic, served in a whole-wheat wrap with diced tomatoes; water	Hearty White Bean Chili (p. 245)*; water	Leftover Sweet Inca Porridge; water or herbal tea
Shake containing chocolate soy protein powder, a sliced banana, ½ cup oats and 1 Tbsp of almond butter; water	Soybean Dinner Loaf (p. 223); steamed broccoli and asparagus; water	Apple; handful raw almonds; water or herbal tea
Clean protein bar; water	Clean-Eating Minestrone Soup (p. 231); slice Ezekiel toast; water	Soy or hemp milk; banana; water or herbal tea
Quinoa mixed with stir-fried black beans, onions, garlic and tomato; water	Rice noodles paired with green onions, cubed tofu, edamame, sesame seeds and tamari sauce; water	Fat-free soy yogurt with berries; water or herbal tea
1 banana with 1 Tbsp almond butter spread on a whole-wheat wrap; water	TVP meatballs with tomato sauce and whole-grain noodles; water	Quinoa Fun Dessert (p. 216); water or herbal tea
Hummus; crudite assortment; water	Light Waldorf Salad (p. 207)***; water	Apple spread with almond butter; water or herbal tea
Hemp protein powder mixed into applesauce; water	Quinoa, chickpeas, tomatoes, and cucumber with tofu, balsamic vinaigrette and olive oil; water	Oatmeal with flaxseed, protein powder and berries; water or herbal tea

GLUTEN-FREE MEAL PLAN

	MORNING START	MIDMORNING BOOSTER	LUNCHTIME REFUEL
DAY 1	Egg-white omelet with mushrooms, tomato, spinach and onion paired with hot brown-rice cereal; water, coffee or green tea	Apple cut into slices with 1 tbsp. almond butter; water	Water-packed tuna with spinach leaves, radishes, carrots, and a squeeze of lemon juice; chick peas; water
DAY 2	Sweet Inca Porridge (pg. 246)** with scrambled egg whites and 1 orange; water, coffee or green tea	Fat-free cottage cheese with mixed berries, flaxseed and millet; water	Leftover brown rice wrapped in a brown-rice wrap spread with yogurt cheese and topped with grilled chicken, tomatoes, and spinach; water
DAY 3	Hard-boiled egg whites; cooked quinoa and mixed berries; water, coffee or green tea	Trail mix (dried apples, cranberries, raisins, almonds, cashews and pumpkin seeds); water	Light Waldorf Salad (pg. 207) with grilled chicken; water
DAY 4	Potato, Rocket and Tomato Frittata (pg. 204); water, coffee or green tea	Sliced carrots, cucumbers, and orange peppers with hummus and gluten-free crackers; water	Fresh spinach with grilled chicken and toasted brown rice wraps cut into triangles; water
DAY 5	Hot rice cereal with mixed berries and vanilla protein powder; water, coffee or green tea	Brown-rice wrap spread with almond butter and wrapped around a banana; water	Leftover grilled chicken sliced onto mesclun greens with chopped carrots, onions, and cucumbers and a squeeze of lemon juice; water
DAY 6	Hot rice milk on top of dry oats**, pumpkin seeds, raisins, chopped almonds, flaxseed, chopped walnuts, cinnamon and nutmeg; water, coffee or green tea	Smoothie with 1 tbsp. all-natural peanut butter with 1 banana, and unsweetened soy milk; water	Tofu sliced onto a brown-rice wrap with hummus, sprouts, cucumbers and tomato; water
DAY 7	Scrambled egg whites with salsa and black beans on a brown-rice wrap; water, coffee or green tea	Sliced apple with 1 tbsp. almond butter; water	Leftover dinner from day 6; water

* check wasabi powder ingredients to be sure it is completely gluten free and use distilled rather than rice vinegar
** purchase uncontaminated oats to ensure they are gluten free
*** read ingredients on chicken broth to ensure there are no gluten fillers
**** check ingredients to ensure there are no gluten fillers

MIDAFTER-NOON MUNCH	DINNER DELIGHT	BEFORE BED IF HUNGRY
Brown-rice cake topped with yogurt cheese and sliced peppers; water	Sesame-Seared Tuna (pg. 220)* with brown rice; water	Fat-free yogurt with sliced strawberries, chopped walnuts and flaxseed; water or green tea
Smoothies with papaya, mango, raspberry, and vanilla protein powder, oats** and flaxseed; water	Roasted carrots, beets, and Brussels sprouts with quinoa and bison tenderloin; water	Vanilla protein powder with strawberries, banana, and kefir; water or green tea
2 celery stalks, rinsed, spread with 1 tbsp. almond butter; water	Swordfish Steaks (pg. 208) with Summertime Risotto (pg. 227)*** water	2 cups air-popped, unbuttered popcorn; nonfat cottage cheese or yogurt; water or green tea
Smoothie with ½ avocado, 1 handful of raspberries and vanilla protein powder; water	Grilled chicken with Black-Eyed Peas and Brown Rice (pg. 237)♦ and steamed green and yellow beans; water ♦ do not use hot sauce	1 apple with 1 handful of almonds; water or green tea
Fat-free cottage cheese with 1 handful of grapes; water	Parchment-Baked Chicken with quinoa, spinach, and roasted zucchini; water	Scrambled egg whites with sliced tomato; water or green tea
Nonfat cottage cheese with chopped apple, cinnamon and nutmeg	Adobo Rubbed Pork (pg. 200)**** with Oven-Baked Brown Rice (pg. 211)**** steamed carrots and broccoli; water	Quinoa Fun Dessert (pg. 216); water or green tea
Chopped cauliflower, broccoli, and cherry tomatoes with carrots; herbed yogurt-cheese dip; water	Lean turkey breast served; quinoa; steamed asparagus and cauliflower; water	Hot brown-rice cereal with unsweetened applesauce and chopped almonds; water or green tea

FAMILY MEAL PLAN
GROCERY LIST

PRODUCE

- ❑ Dates
- ❑ Bananas
- ❑ Tomatoes
- ❑ Mushrooms
- ❑ Apples
- ❑ Pears
- ❑ Celery
- ❑ Raisins
- ❑ Mixed greens
- ❑ Alfalfa sprouts
- ❑ Spinach
- ❑ Onions
- ❑ Cucumbers
- ❑ Blackberries
- ❑ Carrots
- ❑ Red peppers
- ❑ Green peppers
- ❑ Cherry tomatoes
- ❑ Garlic
- ❑ Zucchini
- ❑ Sage, fresh
- ❑ Limes
- ❑ Rosemary, fresh
- ❑ Purple onions
- ❑ Radishes
- ❑ Cilantro
- ❑ Mint leaves
- ❑ Watercress
- ❑ Baking potatoes
- ❑ Porcini mushrooms
- ❑ Shallots
- ❑ Plum tomatoes
- ❑ Lemons
- ❑ Kalamata olives
- ❑ Baby potatoes
- ❑ Kiwi
- ❑ Parsley, fresh
- ❑ Strawberries
- ❑ Raspberries
- ❑ Blueberries
- ❑ Rutabaga
- ❑ Leeks
- ❑ Broccoli
- ❑ Sweet potatoes
- ❑ Arugula
- ❑ Asparagus

DAIRY

- ❑ Eggs
- ❑ Fat-free, sugar-free yogurt (plain and flavored)
- ❑ Fat-free cottage cheese

GRAINS

- ❑ Quinoa
- ❑ Whole-wheat pasta
- ❑ Rolled oats
- ❑ Whole-grain cereal
- ❑ Arborio rice
- ❑ Popcorn (unsalted, unflavored)
- ❑ Whole-wheat couscous
- ❑ Brown rice

SPICES

- ❑ Sea salt
- ❑ Nutmeg
- ❑ Cinnamon
- ❑ Vanilla
- ❑ Ground fennel seed
- ❑ Red pepper flakes

BUTCHER

- ❑ Boneless, skinless chicken breast
- ❑ Lean turkey breast
- ❑ Sea bass
- ❑ Lean beef tenderloin
- ❑ Scallops
- ❑ Salmon fillets

MISCELLANEOUS

- ❑ Bee pollen
- ❑ Green tea
- ❑ Black coffee
- ❑ Wheat germ
- ❑ Vanilla protein powder*
- ❑ Salsa
- ❑ Hummus
- ❑ Vegetable oil
- ❑ Balsamic vinegar
- ❑ Tofu
- ❑ Olive oil
- ❑ Lemon juice
- ❑ Low-sodium soy sauce
- ❑ Grape juice
- ❑ Marsala wine
- ❑ Rice milk
- ❑ Low-sodium chicken broth
- ❑ Unsweetened applesauce
- ❑ Salba crackers
- ❑ Navy beans
- ❑ Clean protein bars

NUTS AND SEEDS

- ❑ Flaxseed
- ❑ Unsalted almonds
- ❑ Almond butter

BAKERY

- ❑ Ezekiel bread
- ❑ Whole-wheat wraps
- ❑ Brown rice cakes

* Use plain protein powder instead and add a dash of vanilla.

VEGAN MEAL PLAN
GROCERY LIST

PRODUCE

- ❏ Green chilies
- ❏ Mushrooms
- ❏ Green onions
- ❏ Pears
- ❏ Alfalfa sprouts
- ❏ Jalapenos
- ❏ Broccoli
- ❏ Asparagus
- ❏ Apples
- ❏ Bananas
- ❏ Leeks
- ❏ Carrots
- ❏ Celery
- ❏ Yukon gold potatoes
- ❏ Zucchini
- ❏ Red onions
- ❏ Green peas
- ❏ Green beans
- ❏ Kale
- ❏ Cabbage (green)
- ❏ Turnip
- ❏ Basil, fresh
- ❏ Parsley, fresh
- ❏ Rosemary, fresh
- ❏ Red grapes
- ❏ Cucumbers
- ❏ Red peppers
- ❏ Mixed greens
- ❏ Tomatoes
- ❏ Onions (yellow)
- ❏ Garlic
- ❏ Lemons
- ❏ Strawberries
- ❏ Mango
- ❏ Raspberries
- ❏ Blueberries
- ❏ Blackberries
- ❏ Plum tomatoes

GRAINS

- ❏ Quinoa
- ❏ Oats
- ❏ Whole-wheat pasta shells (small)
- ❏ Oat bran
- ❏ Brown rice
- ❏ Whole-grain cereal
- ❏ Rice noodles

BAKERY

- ❏ Cinnamon-raisin Ezekiel bread
- ❏ Whole-grain bread
- ❏ Whole-grain wraps

NUTS & SEEDS

- ❏ All-natural peanut butter
- ❏ Almond butter
- ❏ Raw unsalted almonds
- ❏ Flaxseed
- ❏ Walnuts

LEGUMES

- ❏ Black beans
- ❏ White kidney beans
- ❏ Chick peas
- ❏ Navy beans
- ❏ Romano beans
- ❏ Cannelini beans
- ❏ Split peas
- ❏ Lentils

MISCELLANEOUS

- ❏ Unsweetened soy yogurt (plain)
- ❏ Hummus (even better – make your own!)
- ❏ Tofu
- ❏ Low-sodium vegetable broth
- ❏ Salsa
- ❏ Textured vegetable protein

- ❏ Chocolate soy protein powder*
- ❏ Tomato sauce
- ❏ Edamame
- ❏ Rice milk
- ❏ Hemp milk
- ❏ Wheat germ
- ❏ Bee pollen
- ❏ Brown rice cakes
- ❏ Honey
- ❏ Dates
- ❏ Olive oil
- ❏ Unsweetened applesauce
- ❏ Hemp protein powder
- ❏ Clean protein bars
- ❏ Tamari sauce
- ❏ Vanilla soy protein powder*
- ❏ Grape juice
- ❏ Green tea
- ❏ Coffee

*Plain soy protein may be used and add either a dash of vanilla or cocoa powder for flavoring.

GLUTEN-FREE MEAL PLAN
GROCERY LIST

PRODUCE

- Parsnips
- Dates
- Celery
- Red grapes
- Oranges
- Beets
- Brussel sprouts
- Dried, unsweetened apples
- Dried, unsweetened cranberries
- Raisins
- Blackberries
- Papayas
- Garlic
- Red peppers
- Yellow peppers
- Mesclun salad greens
- Mangos
- Blueberries
- Strawberries
- Raspberries
- Green peppers
- Red peppers
- Mixed greens
- Sweet onions
- Jalapeno peppers
- Cilantro, fresh
- Mushrooms
- Tomatoes
- Spinach
- Onions
- Apples
- Radishes
- Carrots
- Lemons
- Bananas
- Parsley, fresh
- Baby new potatoes

- Arugula
- Cherry tomatoes
- Cucumbers
- Orange peppers
- Avocado
- Black-eyed peas
- Butternut squash
- Green beans
- Yellow beans
- Bay leaves
- Watercress
- Mint leaves, fresh
- Cilantro, fresh
- Purple onions
- Limes
- Alfalfa sprouts
- Red onions
- Green onions
- Cilantro, fresh
- Broccoli
- Cauliflower
- Leeks
- Zucchini

DAIRY

- Eggs
- Fat-free, sugar-free yogurt (plain & flavored)
- Fat-free cottage cheese
- Kefir

GRAINS

- Oats*
- Brown rice
- Quinoa
- Wild rice
- Millet
- Popcorn (unsalted, unflavored)
- Gluten-free crackers
- Brown-rice cereal

NUTS & SEEDS

- White sesame seeds
- Black sesame seeds
- Almond butter
- Flaxseed
- Walnuts
- Unsalted almonds
- Unsalted cashews
- Pumpkin seeds
- Pine nuts
- Natural peanut butter

BUTCHER

- Lean turkey breast
- Tuna loin
- Bison tenderloin
- Swordfish steaks
- Water-packed tuna
- Boneless, skinless chicken breasts
- Lean beef tenderloin
- Pork tenderloin

BAKERY

- Brown-rice wraps

SPICES

- Sea salt
- Nutmeg
- Cinnamon
- Vanilla
- Fresh oregano
- Basil, dried
- Thyme, dried
- Paprika
- Chili powder
- Cayenne pepper

MISC.

- Distilled vinegar
- Wasabi powder (check ingredients)
- Sesame oil
- Protein powder**
- Olive oil
- Extra-firm tofu
- Hummus (better to make your own)
- Honey
- Red pepper flakes
- Rice milk
- Soy milk
- Unsweetened applesauce
- Black beans
- Grape juice
- Salsa (check ingredients)
- Green tea
- Coffee

* Purchase uncontaminated oats.

**Use plain protein powder and flavor with a dash of vanilla if desired. Check ingredients.

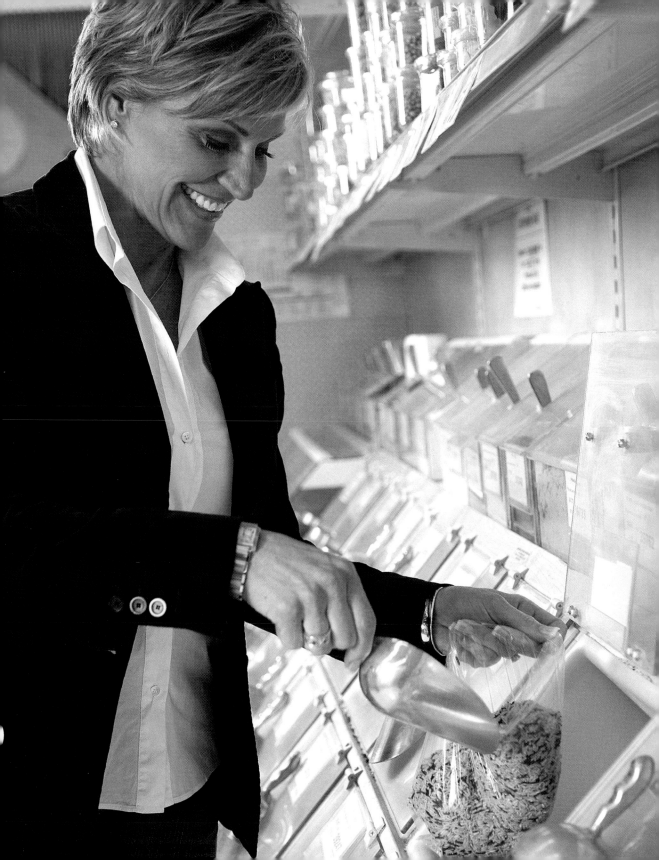

FOOD TRACKER

TIP
Eat every 2-3 hrs starting at breakfast and ending 2-4 hrs before bed. Remember your portion sizes!

	MORNING START	MIDMORNING BOOSTER	LUNCHTIME REFUEL
MON	LP > CC > CC > SUPP > DRINKS >	LP > CC > CC > SUPP > DRINKS >	LP > CC > CC > SUPP > DRINKS >
TUES	LP > CC > CC > SUPP > DRINKS >	LP > CC > CC > SUPP > DRINKS >	LP > CC > CC > SUPP > DRINKS >
WED	LP > CC > CC > SUPP > DRINKS >	LP > CC > CC > SUPP > DRINKS >	LP > CC > CC > SUPP > DRINKS >
THURS	LP > CC > CC > SUPP > DRINKS >	LP > CC > CC > SUPP > DRINKS >	LP > CC > CC > SUPP > DRINKS >
FRI	LP > CC > CC > SUPP > DRINKS >	LP > CC > CC > SUPP > DRINKS >	LP > CC > CC > SUPP > DRINKS >
SAT	LP > CC > CC > SUPP > DRINKS >	LP > CC > CC > SUPP > DRINKS >	LP > CC > CC > SUPP > DRINKS >
SUN	LP > CC > CC > SUPP > DRINKS >	LP > CC > CC > SUPP > DRINKS >	LP > CC > CC > SUPP > DRINKS >

NOTES:

LP = Lean Protein
CC = Complex Carbohydrate

HF = Healthy Fat (olive oil, flaxseed oil, etc)
Supp = Any supplement (vitamins, flax, bee pollen, etc)

MIDAFTER-NOON MUNCH	DINNER DELIGHT	BEFORE BED IF HUNGRY*	HF FOR DAY
LP › CC › CC › SUPP › DRINKS ›	LP › CC › CC › SUPP › DRINKS ›	LP › CC › CC › SUPP › DRINKS ›	
LP › CC › CC › SUPP › DRINKS ›	LP › CC › CC › SUPP › DRINKS ›	LP › CC › CC › SUPP › DRINKS ›	
LP › CC › CC › SUPP › DRINKS ›	LP › CC › CC › SUPP › DRINKS ›	LP › CC › CC › SUPP › DRINKS ›	
LP › CC › CC › SUPP › DRINKS ›	LP › CC › CC › SUPP › DRINKS ›	LP › CC › CC › SUPP › DRINKS ›	
LP › CC › CC › SUPP › DRINKS ›	LP › CC › CC › SUPP › DRINKS ›	LP › CC › CC › SUPP › DRINKS ›	
LP › CC › CC › SUPP › DRINKS ›	LP › CC › CC › SUPP › DRINKS ›	LP › CC › CC › SUPP › DRINKS ›	
LP › CC › CC › SUPP › DRINKS ›	LP › CC › CC › SUPP › DRINKS ›	LP › CC › CC › SUPP › DRINKS ›	

WEEKLY TREAT:

* only if you are hungry!

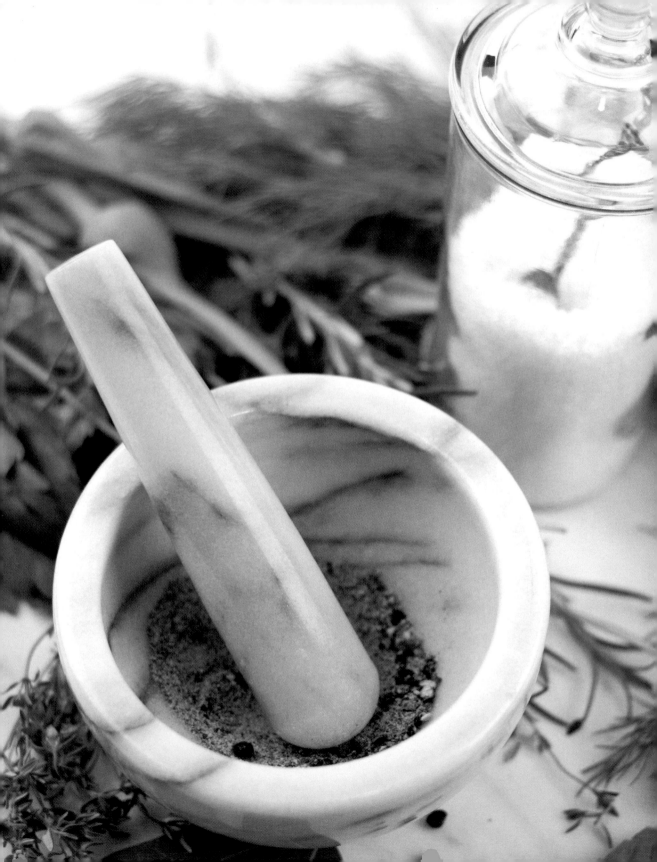

CHAPTER THIRTEEN

EAT-CLEAN
RECIPES

CONTENTS

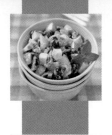
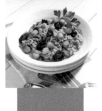
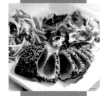

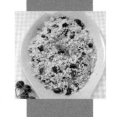
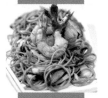
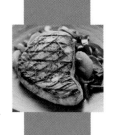
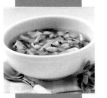

SWEET POTATO
RISOTTO

MAKES 4 SERVINGS

Traditionally, this creamy Italian rice dish requires liquid to be added gradually and stirred constantly – rather labor-intensive for today's time-deprived home cooks. In this version, the rice is stirred only when the sweet potato is added. Serve as a first course, main dish, or side dish with grilled meats or fish.

INGREDIENTS:

2 Tbsp	olive oil
1	onion, chopped
2	cloves garlic, minced
1½ cups	short-grain Italian rice, such as Arborio
4 cups	low-sodium chicken broth, divided
1 Tbsp	white wine vinegar
1 tsp	dried sage
½ tsp	sea salt
½ tsp	dried thyme
¼ tsp	ground black pepper
4 cups	large, bite-size pieces peeled sweet potato
¼ cup	minced fresh parsley *(optional)*

INSTRUCTIONS:

In a large saucepan, heat oil over medium heat. Sauté onion and garlic, stirring, for 2 to 3 minutes. Add rice. Cook, stirring, for another 2 to 3 minutes. Stir in 3 cups of the chicken broth, the vinegar and seasonings. Bring to a boil. Cover and reduce heat to medium-low. Cook for 5 minutes. Stir in sweet potato. Simmer for 15 to 18 minutes, or until sweet potato and rice are tender but still slightly firm. Stir in the remaining cup of chicken broth. The rice should be moist and creamy. Serve immediately, topped with parsley if desired. If rice becomes dry after standing, add a little more chicken broth.

Nutritional information per serving:
170 calories; 5g protein; 2g fat;
31g carbohydrates

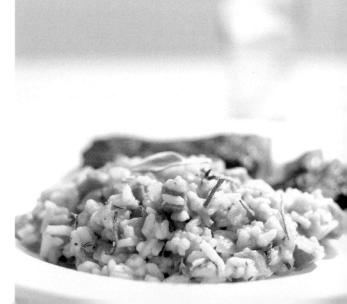

ADOBO-RUBBED PORK TENDERLOIN
with Black-Bean Pico De Gallo

MAKES 4 SERVINGS

PORK
INGREDIENTS:

24 oz	pork tenderloin, trimmed, cut into 3 or 4 oz pieces
6 Tbsp	paprika
2 Tbsp	freshly ground black pepper
2 Tbsp	coarse salt (kosher or sea salt)
1 Tbsp	chili powder
3 pinches	cayenne pepper
½ cup	arugula, loosely packed

PICO DE GALLO
INGREDIENTS:

2 cups	cooked black beans
4 medium	tomatoes, diced
½ cup	red onion, diced
½ cup	green onion, chopped
½ cup	fresh cilantro, chopped
2 Tbsp	jalapeno pepper, minced
2 Tbsp	fresh lemon juice
1 Tbsp	chili powder
½ tsp	salt

INSTRUCTIONS (PORK):

Heat oven to 350°F. Mix paprika, black pepper, salt, chili powder and cayenne pepper together in a bowl. Thoroughly rub both sides of each piece of pork with spice mixture. Heat an oven-safe skillet over medium-high and pan-sear each piece of pork on both sides until golden brown. Pan-searing seals in the meat's juices. Transfer pan to oven until pork is completely done (6 to 8 minutes for each inch of thickness).

INSTRUCTIONS (PICO DE GALLO):

Combine all ingredients. Garnish plates with arugula, add pork in equal portions and sprinkle 1/2 cup Pico de Gallo on the top. Serve.

Nutritional information per serving:
246 calories; 26g protein; 9g fat;
17g carbohydrates

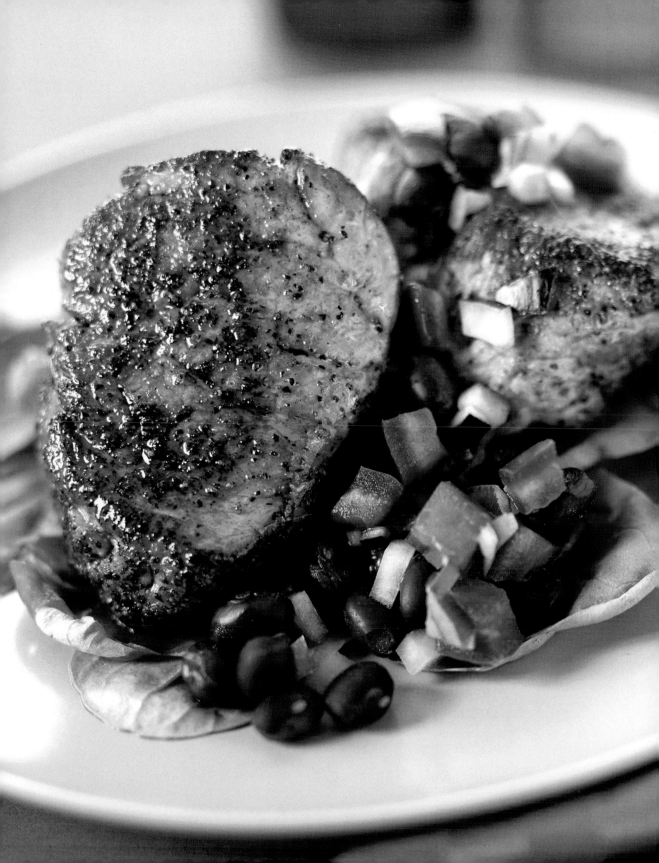

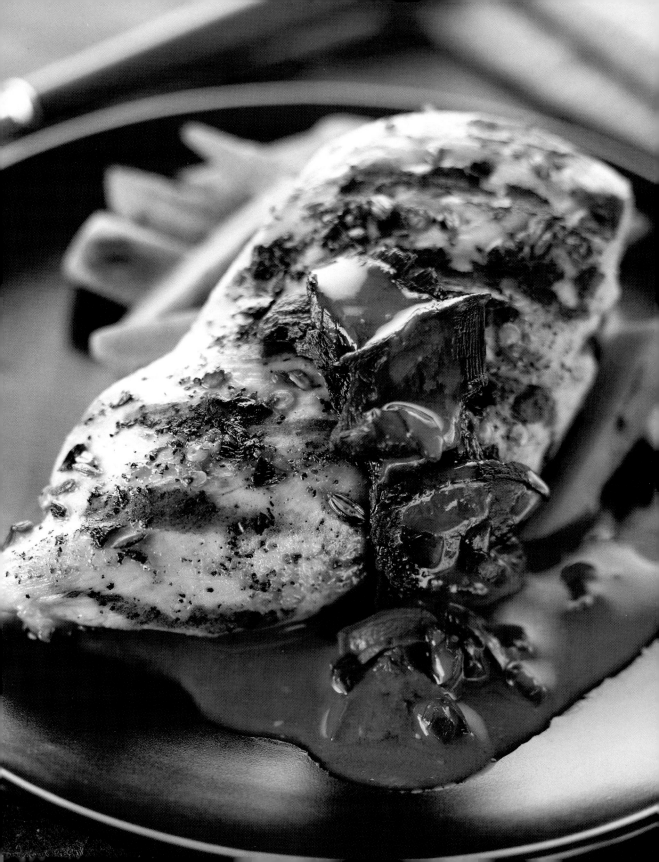

GRILLED BREAST OF CHICKEN MARSALA
with Grilled Carrots

. . . .

MAKES 4 SERVINGS

INGREDIENTS:

4	boneless, skinless chicken breasts (about 6 oz each)
2 tsp	ground fennel seeds
1 tsp	sea salt
½ tsp	freshly ground black pepper
½ tsp	red pepper flakes
16 small	carrots, peeled
3 ½ cups	Marsala wine or low-sodium chicken broth
8	pieces dried porcini mushrooms
2	shallots, thinly sliced
4	cloves garlic, smashed
	Vegetable oil cooking spray
4 Tbsp	nonfat yogurt
4 sprigs	fresh rosemary

INSTRUCTIONS:

Mix fennel, salt, pepper, and red pepper flakes in a bowl. Sprinkle spice mix over chicken and set aside. Place carrots in boiling water for about 4 minutes and remove. Dry on a paper towel. Set aside. Bring Marsala or chicken broth to a low boil in a small saucepan over medium heat. Add mushrooms, shallots, and garlic. Season with salt and pepper. Simmer until sauce reduces, about 20 minutes. Discard garlic and set sauce aside. Coat grill with cooking spray and grill chicken 4 to 6 minutes on each side or until cooked through. Grill carrots about 5 minutes, rotating until charred. Return sauce to stove. Bring to a simmer, then remove from heat and whisk in yogurt. Divide carrots among four plates and top with chicken, sauce and a sprig of rosemary.

Nutritional information per serving (made with Marsala wine) :
688 calories; 48g protein; 31g fat;
62g carbohydrates;

POTATO, ROCKET AND TOMATO FRITTATA

. . . .

MAKES 4 SERVINGS

A frittata can be made quickly in the morning and you can add any ingredients you want to the egg mixture, as long as the vegetables or meat are cooked before the egg is added to the pan. It may seem like a luxury to start the day with a substantial dish like this, but it's actually a great way to get going in the morning. Rocket is a wonderful vegetable common throughout the Mediterranean. It's similar to arugula. It contains iron, folate, calcium, and vitamins C, beta-carotene and K. Potatoes provide vitamin C, potassium and carbohydrate, and tomatoes contain antioxidants, including lycopene, beta-carotene and vitamin C.

INGREDIENTS:

450 g (1lb)	baby new potatoes
1 Tbsp	olive oil
1	garlic clove, crushed
50 g (2 oz)	wild rocket (or arugula)
175 g (6 oz)	cherry tomatoes, halved
8 - 12	egg whites, beaten

Salt and freshly ground black pepper to taste.

INSTRUCTIONS:

Cut potatoes in half, or into chunks if necessary, then cook in a pot of lightly salted boiling water for 8 to 10 minutes. Drain. Heat oil in a non-stick frying pan. Cook the garlic over low heat for one minute. Scatter the potatoes, half the rocket and the cherry tomatoes into the pan. Pour the eggs on top, season well with salt and freshly ground black pepper and cook over a medium heat for about 5 minutes, until almost set. Use a wooden spatula to lift the frittata so any unset egg can travel to the base of the hot pan. When just set on the bottom, place under a preheated broiler for 2 to 3 minutes to set the top. Scatter the remaining rocket overtop and serve.

Nutritional information per serving:
180 calories; 13g protein; 4g fat;
23g carbohydrates;

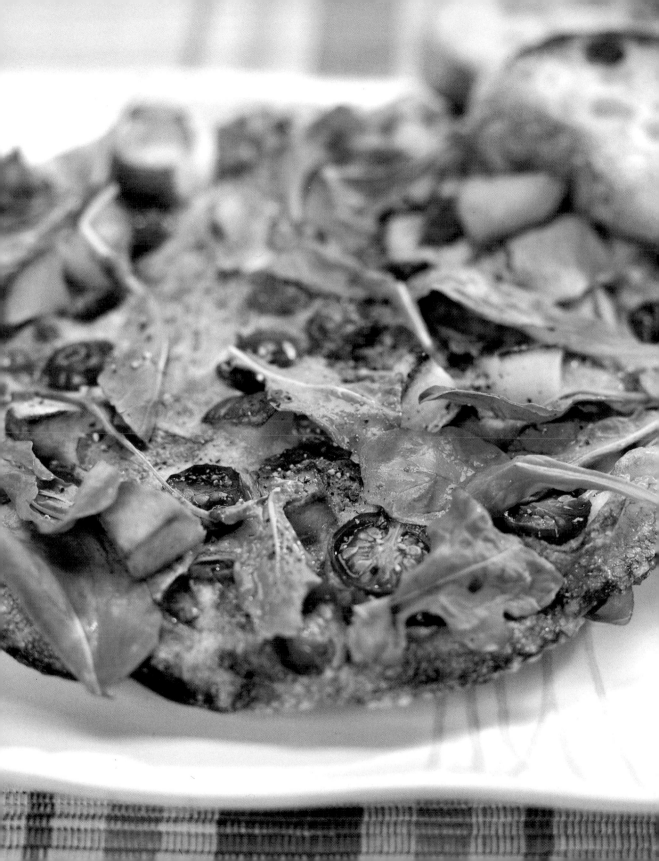

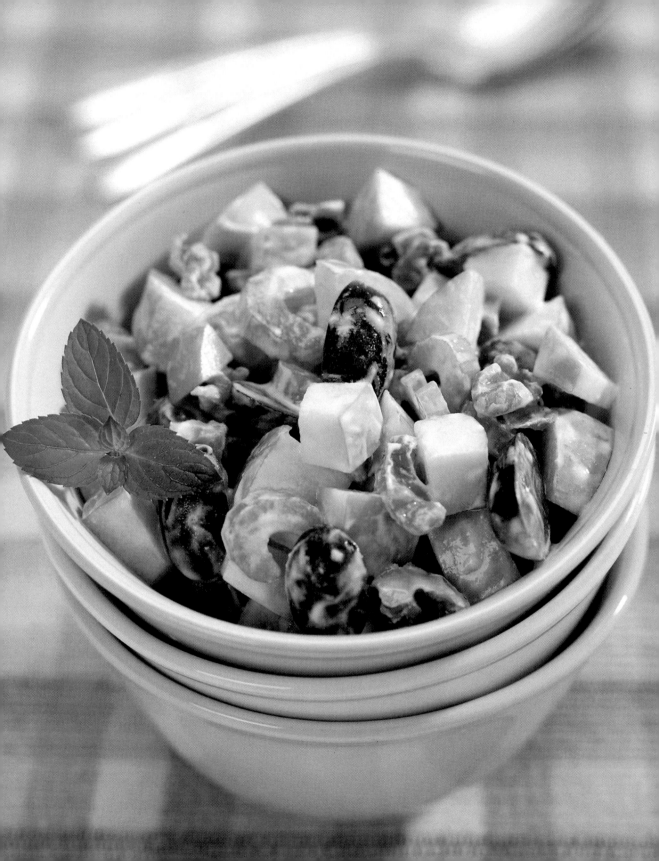

LIGHT WALDORF SALAD

....

MAKES 4 SERVINGS

SALAD INGREDIENTS:

1 cup   diced celery

1 cup   diced crisp apples

½ cup   coarsely chopped walnuts

½ cup   seedless red grapes, halved

DRESSING:

Replace the standard mayonnaise with ½ cup unsweetened, low-fat yogurt mixed with 1 tablespoon lemon juice.

INSTRUCTIONS:

Place all salad ingredients in a large serving bowl. Toss with dressing and keep refrigerated until ready to serve.

Nutritional information per serving:
149 calories; 4g protein; 10g fat;
13g carbohydrates

CHICKEN AND WHITE BEAN SOUP

....

MAKES 12 CUPS

Wondering what to put on the table? Soup is the answer, especially this delicious soup brimming with lean chicken, savory broth and satisfying beans.

INGREDIENTS:

2 tsp   extra virgin olive oil

4   slim leeks, whites and light green centers only, well rinsed, well drained and coarsely chopped

1   large cooking onion, coarsely chopped

1 Tbsp   chopped fresh sage or ½ teaspoon dried sage

6 cups   low-sodium chicken broth or homemade stock

2 cups   water

2 cups   cooked navy beans

2 lbs   chicken breast, grilled and cut into one-inch chunks

8 oz.   package frozen spinach, thawed and partially drained

INSTRUCTIONS:

Heat olive oil in soup pot or Dutch oven. Add drained leeks and chopped onion. Cook until clear and soft, about 5 minutes. Add sage and cook 2 more minutes. Add broth and water and bring to a boil. Add chicken, beans and thawed spinach and continue to cook until all ingredients are uniformly heated.

Nutritional information per serving:
179 calories; 22g protein; 4g fat;
16g carbohydrates

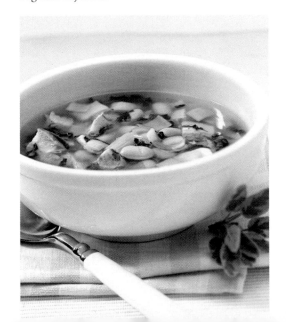

MEDITERRANEAN
SWORDFISH STEAKS

. . . .

MAKES 4 SERVINGS

Swordfish is a little more expensive than cod or haddock. However, for a special occasion it's well worth the extra pennies. If the sun is shining, why not get outside and cook this on the barbecue?

INGREDIENTS:

Juice and finely grated zest of 1 lemon

Juice and finely grated zest of 1 orange

Freshly ground black pepper

1 Tbsp	chopped oregano
4	swordfish steaks, about 175 g (6 oz) each
4 tsp	olive oil
1	garlic clove, crushed
1	red pepper, seeded and cut into fine strips
1	yellow pepper, seeded and cut into fine strips
2	large ripe tomatoes, peeled, seeded and diced
2	oranges, segmented
50 g	bag wild rocket, arugula or mesclun salad greens

INSTRUCTIONS:

Place the lemon and orange zest and juice in a large, shallow dish and stir in the oregano and plenty of black pepper. Cut the swordfish steaks in half diagonally and turn in the marinade to coat thoroughly. Leave at room temperature for 1 hour to marinate. Lift the fish out of the marinade and use 2 teaspoons of the olive oil to brush over both sides.

Heat a large griddle pan until smoking hot and cook the fish for 1 minute. Spin each piece 180 degrees to scorch lines in the opposite direction and cook for another minute. Turn over and repeat on the other side. Remove griddle pan from heat but leave fish to stay hot. Heat remaining oil in a large wok or frying pan. Fry garlic and red and yellow peppers for 2 minutes. Add any remaining marinade and simmer until mixture bubbles. Remove from heat. Stir in diced tomatoes and orange segments. Arrange rocket, arugula or mesclun greens on four serving plates. Lay two pieces of fish on top of each other on the greens, drizzle lemon-orange mixture on top, and serve.

Nutritional information per serving:
304 calories; 34.5g protein; 5g fat;
15g carbohydrate

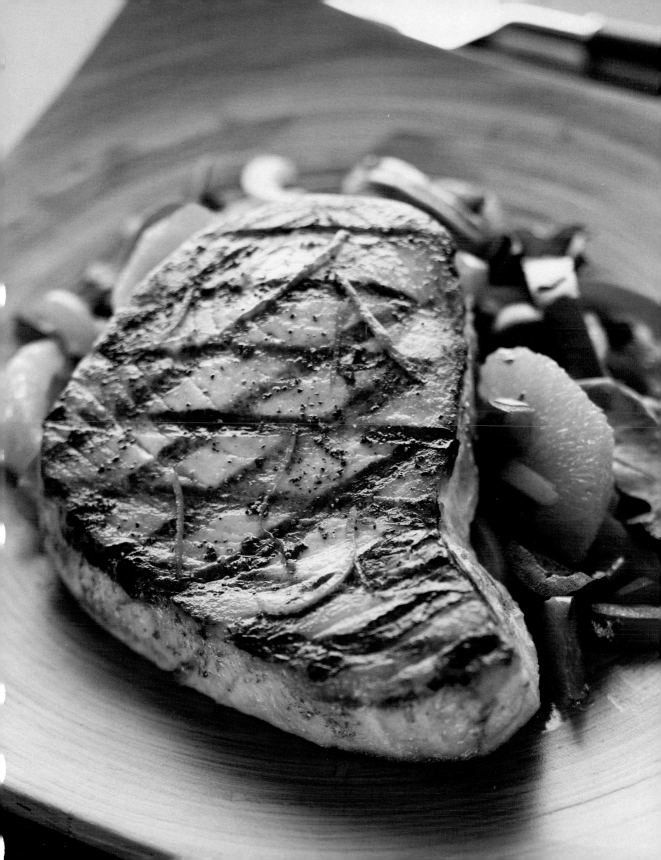

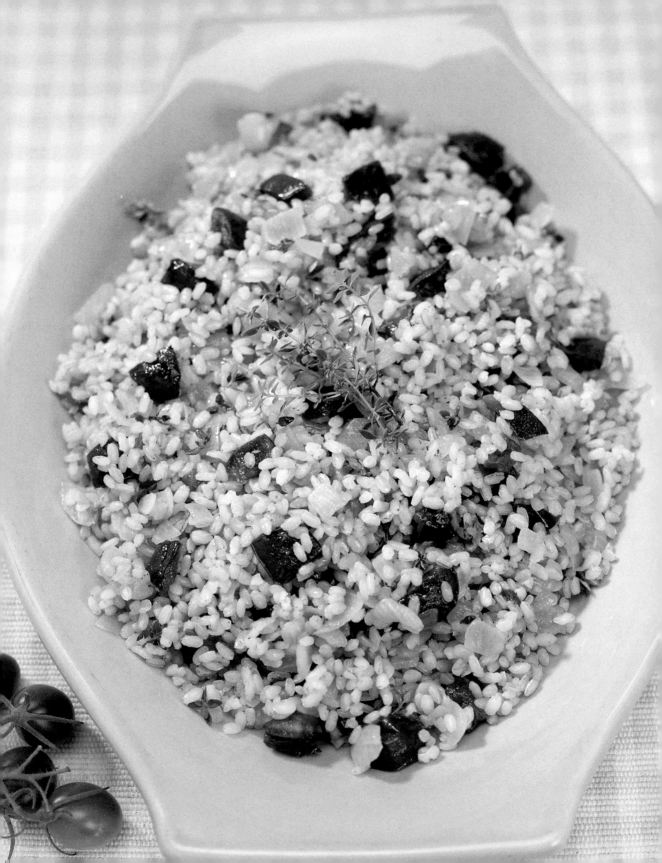

OVEN-BAKED BROWN RICE
with Roasted Tomatoes

. . . .

MAKES 8 SERVINGS

Roasting in the oven makes this rich, creamy rice dish so easy to prepare it requires virtually no attention, yet it develops a consistency similar to a classic risotto.

INGREDIENTS:

8	firm yet ripe plum tomatoes, seeded and coarsely chopped
3 Tbsp	olive oil, best quality
1	yellow onion, chopped
2 cups	short-grain brown rice
1 Tbsp	chopped fresh thyme, plus extra for garnish
4¼ cups	low-sodium chicken stock, heated

Sea salt and freshly ground pepper, to taste

INSTRUCTIONS:

Preheat oven to 400ºF. Line a rimmed baking sheet with aluminum foil. Season the tomatoes with salt and spread them out on the prepared baking sheet. Roast until the edges of the skins are browned but not burned – 10 to 12 minutes. Remove from oven and set aside. Reduce oven temperature to 375ºF. Meanwhile heat oil in Dutch oven or large, heavy ovenproof saucepan with lid. Add the onion and sauté until soft and translucent, about 5 minutes. Add rice and chopped thyme. Season with salt and pepper. Continue to cook, stirring constantly, until the rice is shiny, about 3 minutes. Stir in roast tomatoes. Pour in the hot stock. Stir lightly, cover and bring to a boil. Transfer to oven and continue to cook, covered, until liquid is absorbed – about 40 to 45 minutes. Remove the rice from the oven and fluff with a fork. Transfer to warmed serving bowl. Garnish with thyme sprigs and serve.

Nutritional information per serving:
245 calories; 4g protein; 7g fat;
44g carbohydrates

PARCHMENT-BAKED CHICKEN
with Arugula, Sage, and Rosemary

・・

MAKES 4 SERVINGS *(1 parchment package each)*

INGREDIENTS:

4	(12"x18") parchment sheets
2 cups	arugula leaves, torn
4	(4 oz) skinless, boneless chicken-breast halves
2 tsp	fresh sage, chopped
2 tsp	fresh rosemary, chopped
1 cup	plum tomatoes, chopped
¾ tsp	salt, divided
½ tsp	freshly ground black pepper, divided
4 tsp	olive oil, best quality
4 tsp	kalamata olives, sliced and pitted *(optional)*

Cooking spray

INSTRUCTIONS:

Preheat oven to 450°F. Unfold parchment and coat lightly with cooking spray, leaving a two-inch border. Place ½ cup arugula on one side of the parchment so it touches the fold but not the ungreased border. Place chicken breast over arugula; sprinkle with ½ teaspoon sage and ½ teaspoon rosemary. Top with ¼ cup chopped plum tomato. Sprinkle with one-fourth of the salt and black pepper, and drizzle with 1 teaspoon olive oil. Top with 1 teaspoon sliced olives if desired. Fold paper; seal edges with narrow folds. Repeat with the remaining parchment paper, chicken and other ingredients. Place packets on baking sheets. Bake for 20 minutes or until puffy and lightly browned. To serve, open packets and transfer arugula and chicken breast to plates. Pour juices over top. You can also serve right in packets; carefully transfer to plates and pierce each to allow steam to escape.

Nutritional information per serving:
185 calories; 27g protein; 7g fat;
2g carbohydrates

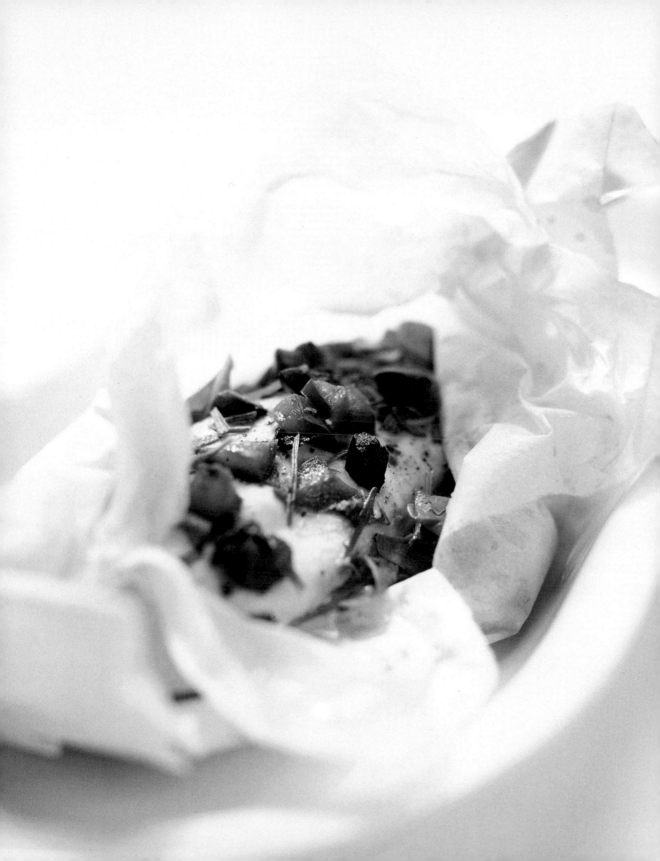

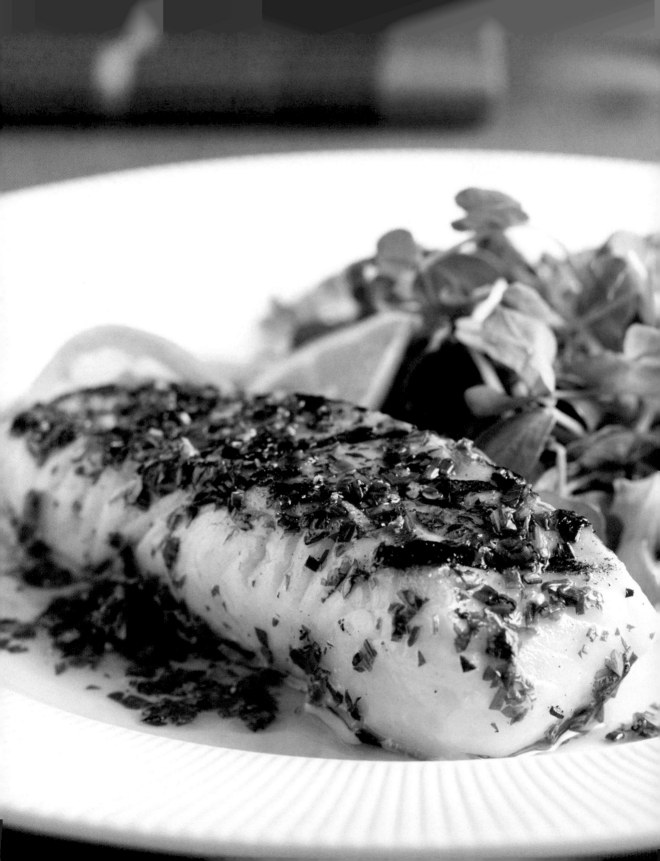

PARCHMENT-BAKED HALIBUT
with Pesto & Vegetables

. . . .

MAKES 4 SERVINGS (*(1 parchment package each)*

In place of halibut, you can use other small, flat, white fish fillets, such as red snapper, sea bass, pompano, striped bass, tilapia or cod.

INGREDIENTS:

4	(12" x 18") sheets parchment paper
4	(6 oz) halibut fillets
4 Tbsp	commercial pesto sauce
1 cup	carrots, shredded (2 medium)
1 cup	zucchini, shredded (1 small)
1 cup	nappa cabbage, shredded
4	cloves garlic, minced
1 tsp	sea salt, divided
1 tsp	freshly ground pepper, divided
4 tsp	olive oil, best quality
4 tsp	low-sodium chicken stock

Cooking spray

INSTRUCTIONS:

Preheat oven to 450°F. Unfold parchment and coat lightly with cooking spray. Leave one two-inch edge ungreased. Place fillet on one side so it touches the fold but not the ungreased edge. Spread 1 table-spoon pesto over fillet and top with 1/4 cup each, carrot, cabbage and zucchini. Sprinkle with one-fourth of the salt and pepper and one minced clove of garlic. Drizzle fillet with 1 teaspoon oil and 1 tea-spoon chicken stock. Fold paper and seal edges with narrow folds. Repeat with the remaining parchment paper, fish, and vegetables. Place packets on baking sheets. Bake for 15 minutes or until puffy and lightly browned. To serve, open packets and transfer the fillets with their vegetable topping to plates. Pour juices over top. Or serve right in packets: carefully transfer to plates and pierce each to allow steam to escape.

Nutritional information per serving:
328 calories; 39g protein; 16g fat;
6g carbohydrates

QUINOA FUN DESSERT

MAKES 3 SERVINGS

INGREDIENTS:

1 cup   quinoa
4 or 5   dates, chopped
2 cups   grape juice
½ cup   raisins

INSTRUCTIONS:

Combine all ingredients in a pot and cook mixture together on medium heat. Serve hot or cold. Sliced frozen banana can be added before serving.

Nutritional information per serving:
435 calories; 9g protein; 3.5g fat;
96g carbohydrates

LEEK & POTATO SOUP

MAKES 10 CUPS

A simple way to boost the immune system and fight disease is to consume more foods from the onion family such as leeks. Loaded with phytonutrients, onions ward off early signs of aging and fight infection.

INGREDIENTS:

6   leeks, whites only, well rinsed and drained, coarsely chopped

4   medium baking potatoes

1 Tbsp   extra virgin olive oil

¼ cup   chopped onion

3   cloves garlic, minced

8 cups   low-sodium, low-fat chicken broth or homemade stock

INSTRUCTIONS:

Wash leeks thoroughly. Cut into one-inch pieces. Place in a colander and rinse again. Drain. Peel potatoes and cut into one-inch chunks. In a large saucepan or Dutch oven, heat olive oil. Add leeks, potatoes, onion and garlic. Cook for 5 to 10 minutes, until soft. Add stock to saucepan and bring to a boil. Once mixture has come to a full boil, reduce heat and cook for another 30 minutes until all vegetables are soft. Purée soup in a blender or food processor.

Nutritional information per serving:
92 calories; 6g protein; 3g fat; 11g carbohydrates

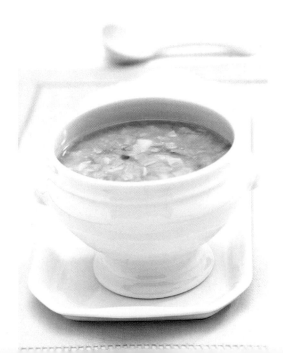

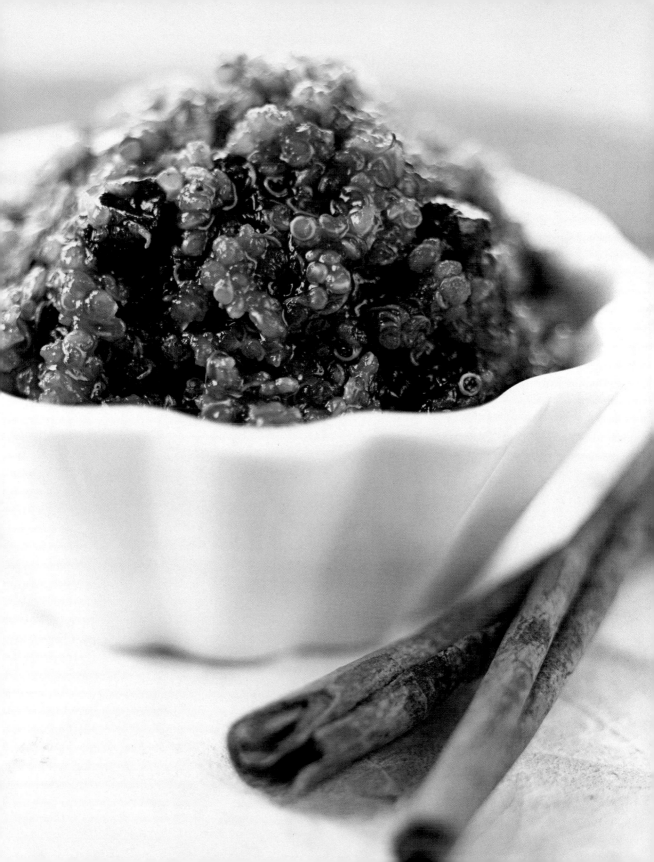

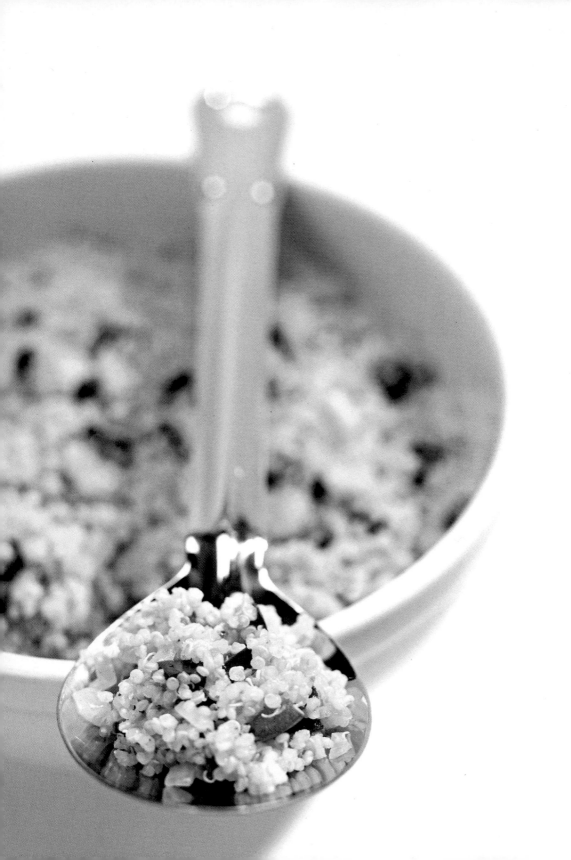

QUINTESSENTIAL
QUINOA

MAKES 8 SERVINGS

This is a perfect recipe as an introduction to healthy eating, even for the hardcore junk-food addict. It tastes simply scrumptious.

INGREDIENTS:

2 Tbsp	olive oil, best quality
4	medium yellow onions, chopped
3	garlic cloves, minced
½ tsp	sea salt
1	large red pepper, chopped
2 cups	rinsed quinoa
4 cups	water
2	vegetarian soup-stock cubes or low-sodium chicken-flavored cubes

INSTRUCTIONS:

Add finely chopped onion, minced garlic and salt to olive oil in wok and sauté until onions are slightly brown. Add chopped red pepper and continue to sauté until onions are caramelized. Add water, stock cubes and rinsed quinoa. Bring mixture to a simmer. Stir once after 5 minutes, then simmer for another 35 minutes or until water has been cooked in. Fluff quinoa mixture lightly with a fork.

Nutritional information per serving:
220 calories; 6g protein; 6g fat;
37g carbohydrates

SESAME-SEARED TUNA
with Vegetable Slaw

. . . .

MAKES 4 SERVINGS

INGREDIENTS:

Slaw

2	carrots, peeled
2	parsnips, peeled
2 each	green and red bell peppers, cored and seeded
1	small sweet onion
1	jalapeno pepper, cored (and seeded for less heat)
2	Tbsp chopped fresh cilantro

Dressing

½ cup	nonfat yogurt
½ cup	rice vinegar

Sea salt and white pepper

Seeds from ½ vanilla bean

Tuna

½ cup	white sesame seeds
½ cup	black sesame seeds
1 Tbsp	wasabi powder (found at Asian grocery stores)
1 Tbsp	sesame oil
2 pieces	tuna loin (about 8 oz each), cut in half

Greens (such as baby spinach)

Vegetable-oil cooking spray

INSTRUCTIONS:

Slaw

Attach grating blade to food processor. Julienne each vegetable and set aside. Combine dressing ingredients in a bowl. Add vegetables and cilantro. Mix gently. Let rest for 30 minutes.

. . . .

Tuna

Combine sesame seeds and wasabi in a bowl; season with salt and pepper. Heat large nonstick pan over high heat. Coat pan with cooking spray then drizzle in oil. Salt tuna lightly, then coat with the sesame-wasabi mixture. Reduce heat to medium. Sear tuna until lightly browned, about 2 minutes. Flip, then cook 2 minutes more. Remove from heat and let rest for a few minutes. Divide slaw among 4 plates, top with tuna and garnish with greens.

Nutritional information per serving:
458 calories, 33.5g protein; 14.8g fat (2.3g saturated); 50.6g carbohydrates

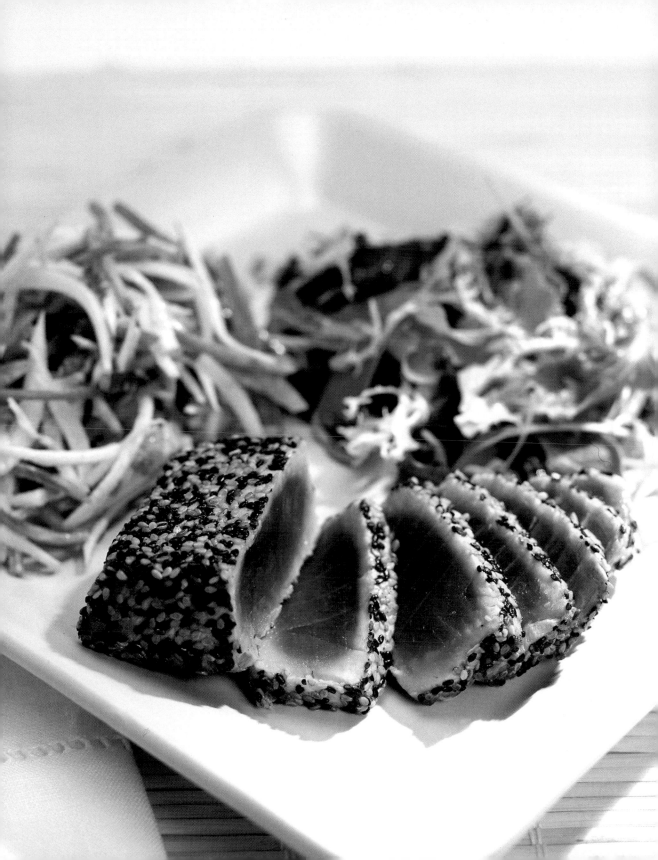

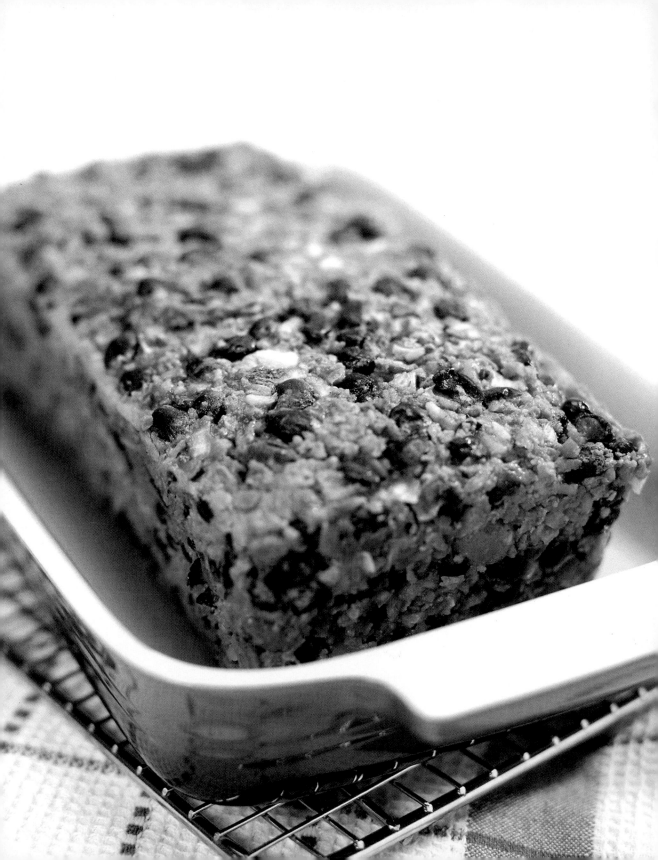

SOYBEAN DINNER LOAF

. . . .

MAKES 8 - 10 SERVINGS

INGREDIENTS:

1 cup   textured vegetable protein

2 cups   Mexican-style tomato sauce

2 cups   cooked black beans, rinsed and drained

2   egg whites, lightly beaten

¼ cup   raisins

1 small yellow onion, chopped

1 small fresh jalapeno pepper, seeded and minced

¾ cup   combination of oat bran and cooked brown rice

½ cup   cilantro, chopped

Sea salt and freshly ground black pepper

INSTRUCTIONS:

Preheat oven to 350°F. Mix all ingredients in a large bowl with clean bare hands. Prepare a 9" x 5" loaf pan with non-stick cooking spray. Pack loaf mixture in pan. Cover with aluminum foil and bake for 20 to 30 minutes or until set. Remove from heat and let stand for 12 minutes before serving.

Nutritional information per serving:
181 calories; 21g protein; 2g fat;
29g carbohydrates

STIR-FRIED BOK CHOY
with Noodles

. . . .

MAKES 1 SERVING

You can also stir-fry a protein source such as prawns or chicken. If you do so, add to the stir-fry with the mushrooms and bok choy.

INGREDIENTS:

25 g (1oz)	whole-grain angel-hair pasta
1 Tbsp	soy sauce
1 Tbsp	teriyaki sauce
2 Tbsp	dry sherry
1 tsp	minced ginger
2 tsp	olive oil
125 g (4 oz)	bok choy, sliced
125 g (4 oz)	shiitake mushrooms, thickly sliced
2	spring onions, sliced

INSTRUCTIONS:

Cook pasta in a pan of lightly salted boiling water for 5 minutes. Drain well and set aside. Mix soy and teriyaki sauces, sherry and ginger in a small bowl. Heat oil in a large frying pan or wok. Add bok choy and mushrooms, and stir-fry for 2 minutes. Pour in the sauce, add the pasta and stir-fry for a further 2 minutes. Add spring onions, mix well and serve.

Nutritional information per serving:
219 calories; 8.5g protein; 7.2g fat;
23g carbohydrate

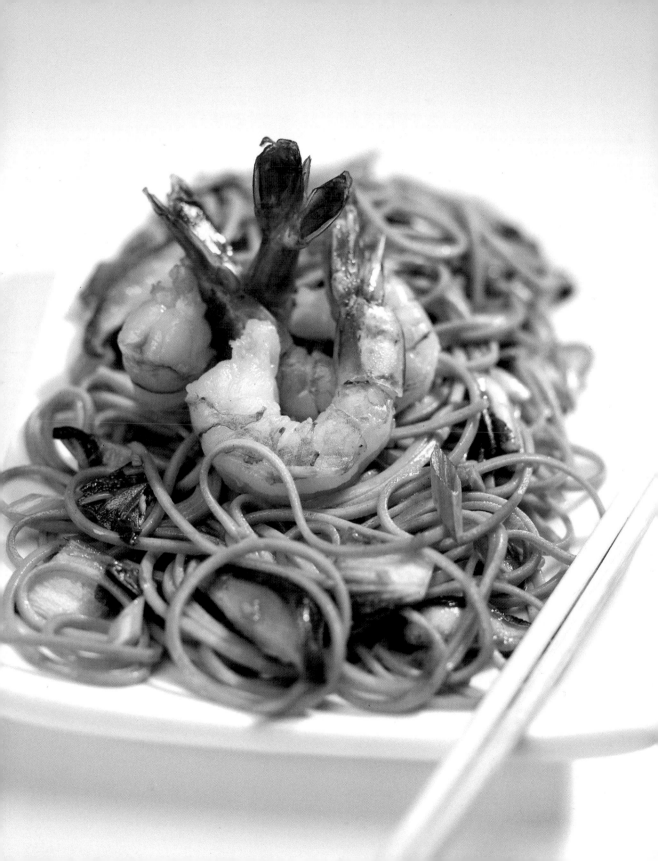

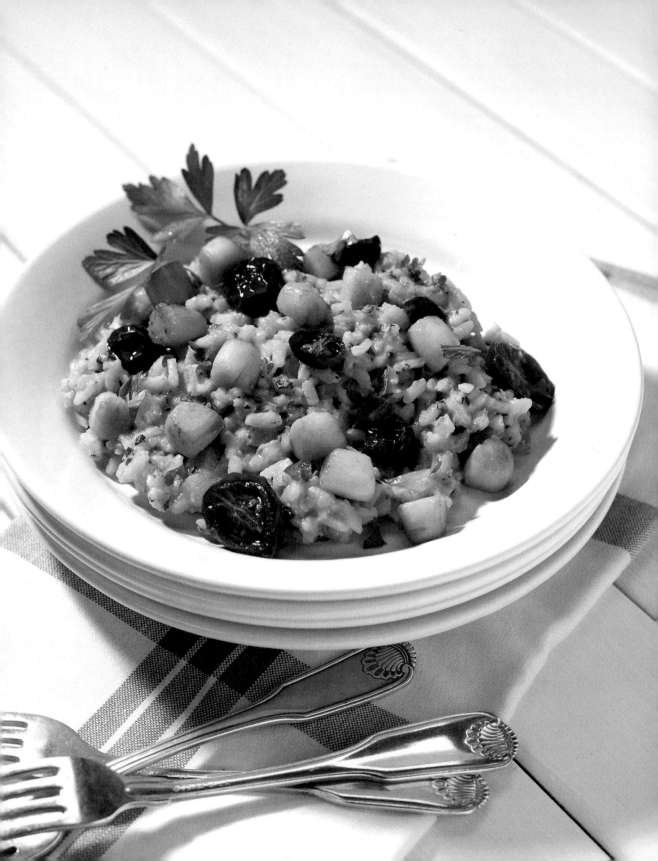

SUMMERTIME RISOTTO

MAKES 6 SERVINGS

INGREDIENTS:

1 pint   cherry tomatoes, roasted

4 Tbsp   olive oil, best quality

1 tsp   garlic, minced

1 small onion, diced

2 cups   diced zucchini

¼ cup   fresh lemon juice

1 pound Arborio rice

3-4 cups fat-free chicken broth

1 pound scallops, washed

salt

pepper

1 bunch parsley, chopped (optional)

INSTRUCTIONS:

Roasted tomatoes – Toss tomatoes in 2 teaspoons oil with a pinch of salt and pepper. Place on non-stick baking sheet and bake 1 hour at 250°F.

Zucchini purée – In a medium pan, heat 1 teaspoon oil over medium heat. Add garlic and half the onion and cook until translucent. Add zucchini and cook 5 minutes. Place all these ingredients in a blender. Add lemon juice and 1 tablespoon oil and purée. Add salt and pepper to taste. Set aside.

Risotto – Heat 1 tablespoon oil in medium pot on medium heat and sauté remaining onion until translucent. Add rice and stir to coat. Add broth 1 cup at a time until absorbed, stirring continually for 20 minutes or until rice is tender (add more broth if necessary). Once rice is cooked, stir in zucchini purée. Set aside.

Scallops – Heat 1 tablespoon oil in small pan. Season scallops with salt and pepper and cook both sides until lightly browned. Add tomatoes and sauté 5 minutes. Place risotto on plate and top with scallops, tomatoes and parsley.

Nutritional information per serving:
488 calories; 16g protein; 11g fat;
68.5g carbohydrates

THAI BEEF SALAD

MAKES 6 SERVINGS

BEEF INGREDIENTS:

12 cups	water
1½ pounds	lean beef tenderloin
3	bay leaves

SALAD INGREDIENTS:

3 bunches	watercress, washed and dried, tough stems and wilted leaves removed
1½ cups	fresh mint leaves, washed and picked over
1½ cups	fresh cilantro leaves, washed and picked over
2 bunches	red radishes, washed and sliced thinly, tops removed
1 medium	purple onion, thinly sliced
2 Tbsp	lemon zest, cut into thin strips

DRESSING

¼ cup	extra virgin olive oil, best quality
¼ cup	freshly squeezed lime juice
1 Tbsp	low-sodium soy sauce

Red pepper flakes to desired spiciness

Sea salt and freshly ground black pepper

INSTRUCTIONS:

Combine all salad ingredients in a large bowl. Cover with a damp kitchen towel and refrigerate until ready to serve.

In large soup kettle bring 12 cups water to a full boil. Add 3 bay leaves and 1½ pounds lean beef tenderloin, all fat removed. Cover meat and simmer for 20 minutes till meat is medium rare. Remove beef from kettle. Cover and let stand for 15 minutes.

Slice tenderloin in 1/2-inch-thick strips. Remove salad from fridge. Toss tenderloin and dressing into salad and serve.

Nutritional information per serving:
332 calories; 24g protein; 23g fat;
10g carbohydrates

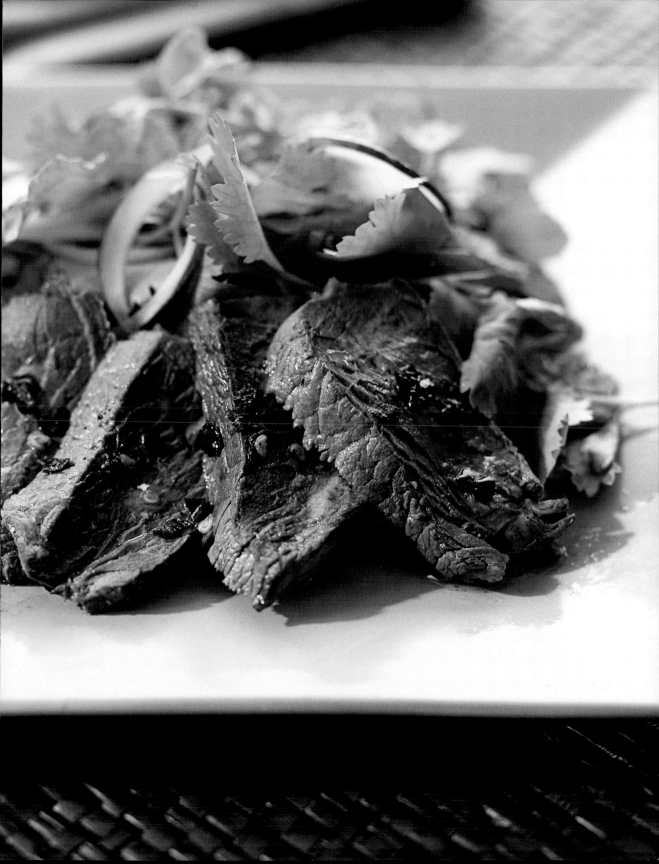

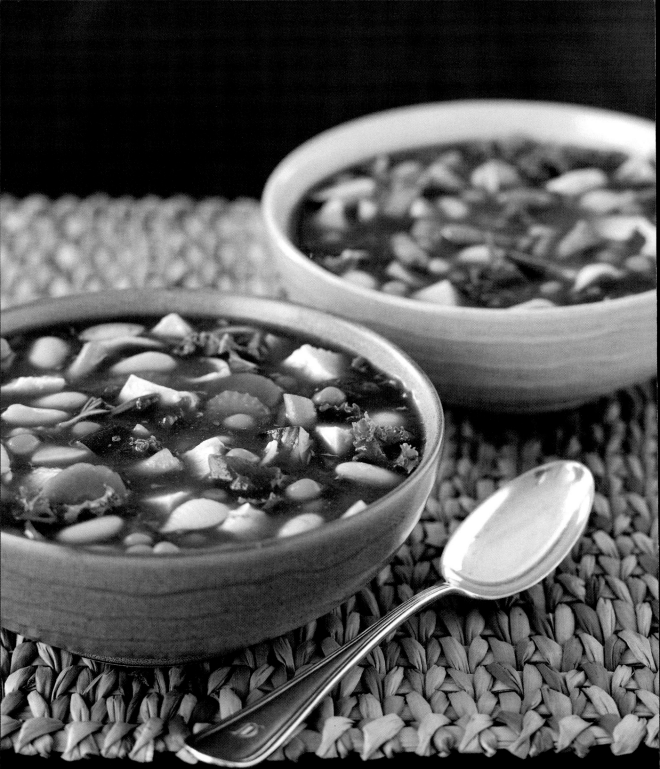

CLEAN-EATING MINESTRONE SOUP

MAKES 24 CUPS *(Freezes Well)*

Minestrone is an ideal Clean-Eating soup. Brimming with superfoods, it satisfies the stomach and the soul. Simmer up a batch and let it feed you.

INGREDIENTS:

1	leek, whites only, halved, rinsed and sliced
2 cups	blanched diced tomatoes
3	carrots, peeled and sliced into rounds
1	onion, cut into one-inch chunks
½	red onion, cut into one-inch chunks
4	stalks of celery, threads removed, chopped
2	Yukon Gold potatoes, washed, skin on, cut into one-inch chunks
2	zucchini, diced
4 oz (½ cup)	cannelini beans
8 oz (1 cup)	green peas
3	cloves of garlic, minced
4 Tbsp	olive oil, best quality
¼ pound	green beans, trimmed
½ pound	kale or spinach, rinsed, drained and chopped
½	green cabbage, shredded
1	small turnip, peeled and diced
2 Tbsp	fresh basil
2 Tbsp	fresh parsley
2 Tbsp	fresh rosemary
½ cup	small pasta shells
2 liters (8 cups)	low-sodium vegetable juice
16 cups	low-sodium chicken, beef or vegetable stock
2	large chicken breasts or one turkey breast, cooked and diced, *optional*

Sea salt and pepper

INSTRUCTIONS:

Prepare the dried beans by bringing 2 liters (8 cups) of water to a boil in a large saucepan. Add the beans and bring the water to a boil. Remove from heat and let soak in the pan overnight. Drain the beans, reserving the liquid. Purée half the beans in a food processor or blender. Stir the purée and the remaining whole beans into the soup. In a large soup pot, heat olive oil. Add all fresh vegetables except tomatoes and spinach. Cook for a few minutes until lightly colored. Add cooked meat if using. Add seasonings, green beans, chicken stock and tomatoes. Simmer for 2 hours. Add pasta shells and cook for another 30 minutes. Toss spinach into pot just before serving.

Nutritional information per serving:
(with 2 chicken breasts)
126 calories; 6g protein; 3.5g fat;
19g carbohydrates

BLUEBERRY PEACH COBBLER SMOOTHIE

MAKES 1 SMOOTHIE

INGREDIENTS:

1 scoop	plain or vanilla protein powder
½ cup	skim milk
½ cup	blueberries
1 sliced	peach
½ cup	plain, nonfat yogurt
1 tsp	Sucanat
½ tsp	vanilla

Nutritional information per serving:
296 calories; 32g protein; 1.4g fat;
38g carbohydrates

INSTRUCTIONS:

Purée all ingredients. You may need to pulse a few times. Slowly add a small amount of skim milk while blending if the mixture is too thick. If you want to make this more "cobbler" like, then place the peach and blueberries in a small saucepan with a tablespoon or two of water. Cook till the fruit becomes slightly syrupy, and then purée it in the blender with the rest of the ingredients. Mmmmm, dessert!

TURKEY MEATBALLS

MAKES 4 LARGE MEATBALLS

INGREDIENTS:

⅓ cup	finely chopped yellow or sweet onion
⅓ cup	finely chopped green bell pepper
¼ cup	water or low-sodium chicken broth
1 pound	ground lean turkey breast, no skin
¼ cup	oat bran
1 tsp	dried celery flakes
½ tsp	ground sage
¼ tsp	ground marjoram
¼ tsp	dried thyme
1 tsp	Worcestershire sauce
¼ tsp	ground black pepper
1	egg white

Nutritional information per serving:
160 calories, 30g protein, 1.8g fat,
5g carbohydrates

INSTRUCTIONS:

In a small skillet, heat water or chicken broth and sauté the onion and green pepper until translucent. In a mixing bowl, combine remaining ingredients. Add cooked onion and pepper. Coat clean hands with a little olive oil and mix thoroughly. Shape into four equal-sized meatballs and place on a cookie sheet. Place in preheated 350°F oven and bake until browned – about 20 minutes.

(Note: *You could also use lean ground chicken breast)*

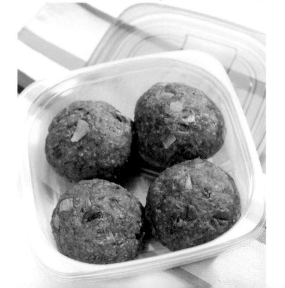

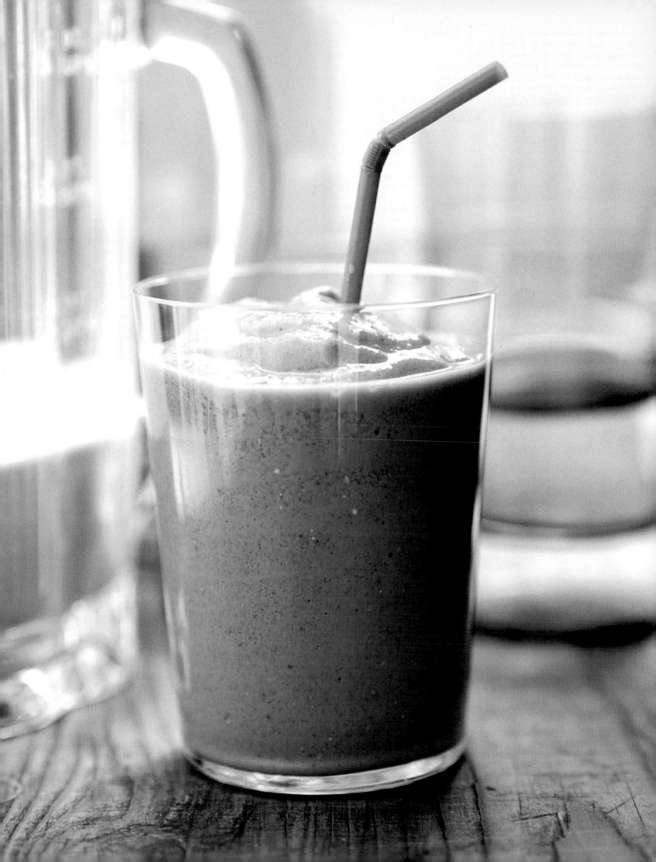

ROASTED GARLIC &
SWEET POTATO SOUP

MAKES 10 CUPS

Roasted garlic adds superb flavor to any soup. Roasting whole heads of garlic in the oven is much simpler than it sounds and removes the bitterness. Garlic helps reduce blood pressure, reduces the risk of heart disease and fights cancer.

INGREDIENTS:

6	large sweet potatoes
1	large cooking onion, chopped
1 Tbsp	extra virgin olive oil
1 head	roasted garlic
6 cups	reduced-salt chicken broth or bouillon
1 or 2 cups of water	

INSTRUCTIONS:

Preheat oven to 350°F. Slice potatoes in half lengthwise. Rub cut surfaces with olive oil and place cut side down on a baking sheet. On the same baking sheet, place a whole bulb of garlic and drizzle with more olive oil. Bake uncovered in center of oven until the sweet potatoes are soft, about 45 minutes.

Meanwhile heat olive oil in a sauté pan. Add chopped onion and sauté until clear and soft. Place in food processor. Remove half the potato pulp from the sweet potatoes and place in a food processor. Squeeze the roasted garlic into the food processor with sweet potato pulp. Run the food processor until a smooth purée forms. Place purée into a large saucepan and add remaining puréed potato pulp. Add broth and water until desired consistency. Cook on medium until thoroughly heated.

Nutritional information per serving:
99 calories; 3.5g protein; 1.5g fat;
18g carbohydrates

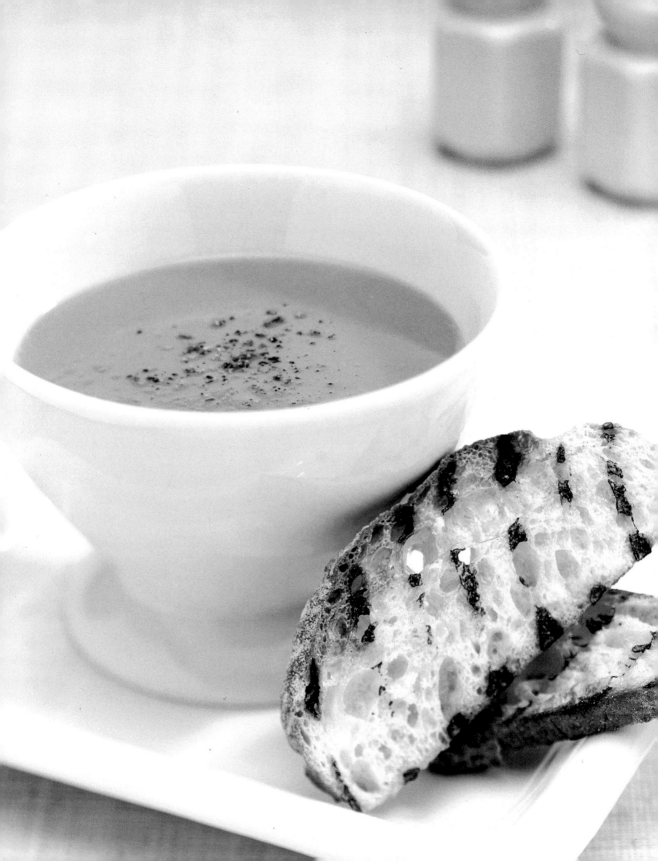

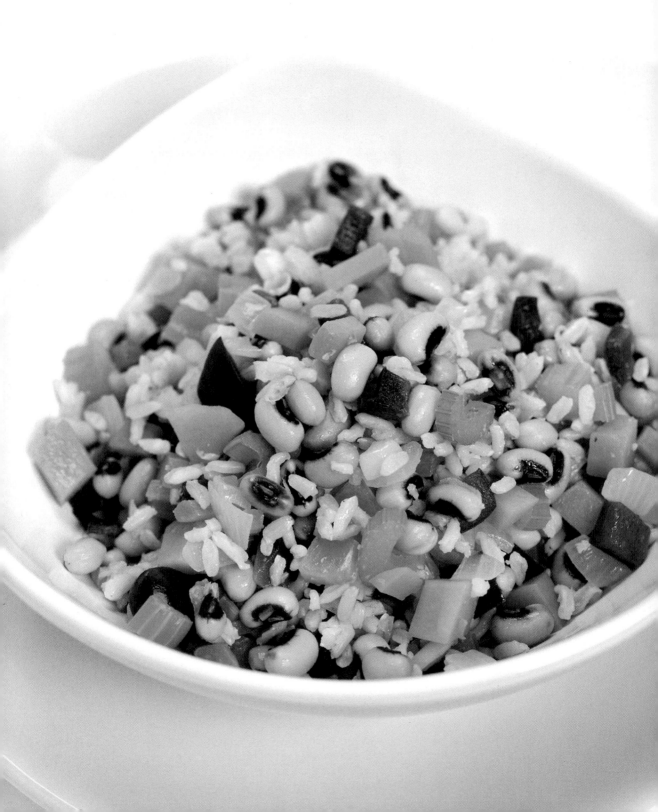

BLACK-EYED PEAS AND
BROWN RICE

. . . .

MAKES 6 SERVINGS

This grain and legume mixture is a true Clean-Eating dish, loaded with protein and fiber. Buy frozen, cooked black-eyed peas, or start with the dried legume and cook up a batch yourself, freezing any extra for future meals.

INGREDIENTS

4 cups	cooked, cold, long-grain brown rice
1 ¼ cups	water
1	onion, chopped
2	celery stalks, chopped
2	garlic cloves, minced
¼ tsp	freshly ground pepper
3 cups	cooked black-eyed peas
1	butternut squash, about one pound, peeled, seeded, and cut into cubes
1	red bell pepper, stemmed, seeded and finely chopped
½ tsp	hot pepper sauce

INSTRUCTIONS:

Put rice in a large bowl. Gently separate the grains and break apart any lumps. In a large frying pan, bring the water, onion, celery, garlic and pepper to a boil, stirring frequently. Add the black-eyed peas and squash and return to a boil, again stirring frequently. Reduce to low, cover and simmer, stirring occasionally, until the peas and squash are tender and most of the water has evaporated, about 20 minutes. Add the rice, bell pepper and hot-pepper sauce. Simmer, stirring and tossing frequently, until heated through, about 5 minutes. To serve, transfer to a bowl.

Nutritional information per serving:
268 calories; 11g protein; 1g fat; 59g carbohydrates.

STELLAR LEGUME SOUP

. . . .

MAKES 16 CUPS

Legumes are a superior source of protein, complex carbohydrates and fiber. Complex carbohydrates are slow burning and help you feel full longer. Bean soups make a delicious meal, especially with a piece of hearty whole-grain bread.

INGREDIENTS

1¼ cups	mixed dried beans, including black beans, navy beans, kidney beans and Romano beans
¼ cup	lentils
¼ cup	split peas
¼ cup	barley
Water	
2	cooking onions, coarsely chopped
3	large carrots, peeled and coarsely chopped
4-5	celery stalks, coarsely chopped
10 cups	low-sodium chicken broth
3 cups	stewed plum tomatoes
¼ tsp	dried thyme leaves, crumbled
1	bay leaf
½ tsp	coarsely ground black pepper
1	sweet red bell pepper, seeded and coarsely chopped
2-3	garlic cloves, roasted
½ cup	chopped fresh parsley

INSTRUCTIONS:

Put dried beans in a large saucepan and cover with generous amounts of water. Bring to a rolling boil over high heat, uncovered. Remove from heat and cover. Let sit for one hour. Drain. Rinse barley, lentils and split peas. Drain. In large sauté pan, add onions, celery and carrots. Add broth, tomatoes plus their juice, seasonings, beans and lentils, split peas and barley. Boil. Cover and reduce heat to low. Cook, stirring occasionally, until beans and vegetables are tender – approximately 2 hours. Add chopped bell pepper and roasted garlic. Simmer for another 5 minutes. Add chopped parsley and serve.

Nutritional information per serving:
102 calories; 7g protein; 1g fat;
18g carbohydrates.

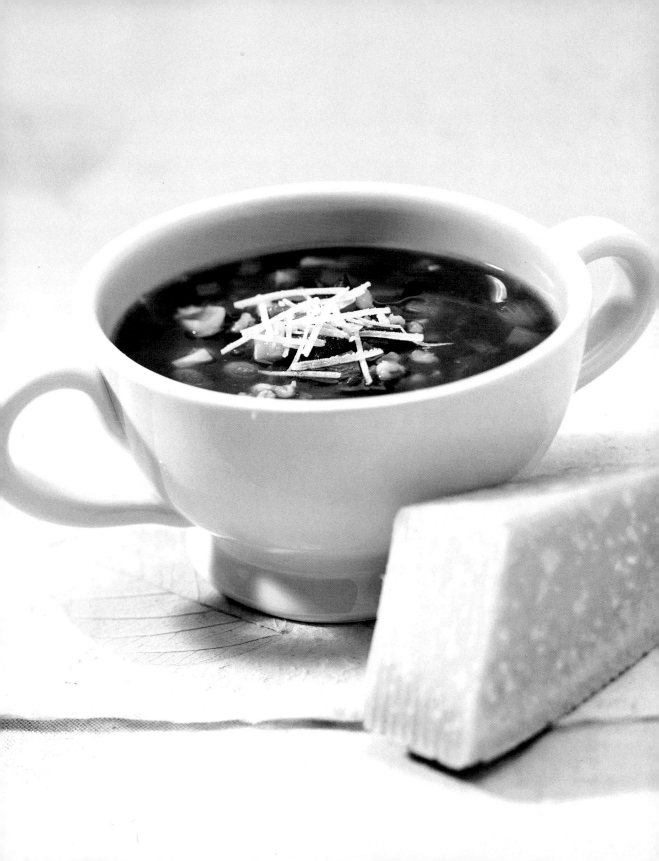

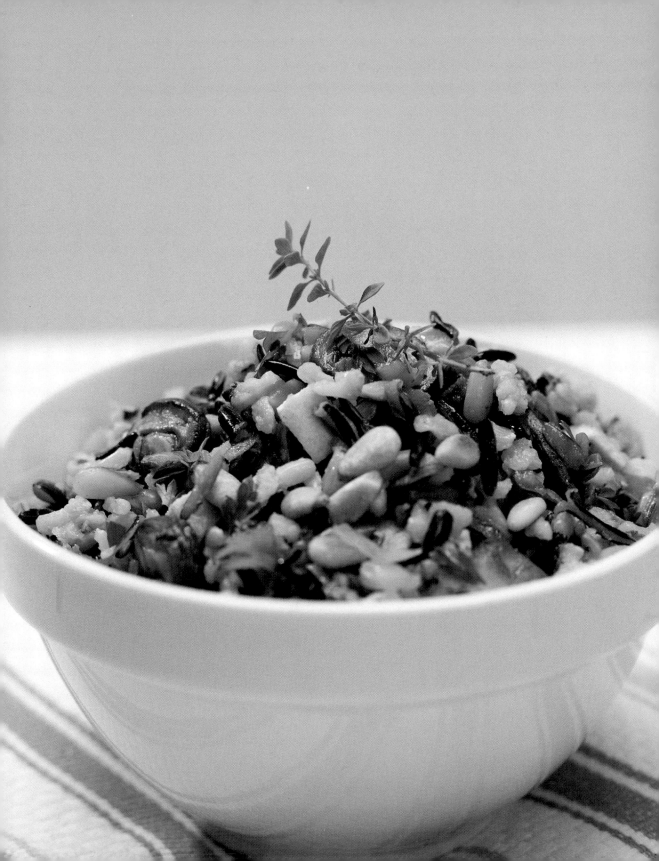

FESTIVE WILD RICE

Deeply colored varieties of rice hold immense nutritional value. First Nations peoples of North America enjoyed wild rice, not really rice but rather a variety of corn, in many of their staple foods. Brown or whole-grain rice is known to regulate blood-sugar levels while white rice does not.

INGREDIENTS

1 cup	long-grain brown rice
1 cup	wild rice
½ cup	pine nuts
6 cups	water or low-sodium chicken stock
½ cup	sliced mushrooms
½	onion, chopped
1	block extra-firm tofu, cubed
2 Tbsp	low-sodium soy sauce
½ tsp	each basil, thyme and sea salt

Fresh parsley for garnish

INSTRUCTIONS:

Preheat oven to 350ºF. Wash and rinse rice. Toast pine nuts over medium heat in a frying pan. Nuts should be golden. Prepare casserole dish with cooking spray. Place water and rice in casserole dish. Arrange all other ingredients on top of rice. Don't mix them in. Cover and bake until all the water is absorbed. This will take about 1 to 1 1/2 hours. Garnish with the parsley and serve.

Nutritional information per serving:
355 calories; 15g protein; 13g fat;
48g carbohydrates.

TOMATO AND ROASTED
GARLIC SOUP

. . . .

MAKES 12 CUPS

The flavors of this soup – garlic, tomato, basil and oregano – when combined, taste like summer in a bowl. Chockfull of goodness and luscious cancer-fighting tomatoes, this soup will satisfy hunger and sustain you through a busy day.

INGREDIENTS

1 head garlic

1 tsp   extra virgin olive oil, divided

Salt and pepper

1 cup   chopped onion

1 cup   chopped celery

8 cups stewed tomatoes, including juice

1   bay leaf

2 tsp   dried oregano

2 tsp   dried basil

1 cup   water

1 tsp   dried thyme

INSTRUCTIONS:

Preheat oven to 400ºF. Remove loose, papery skins from garlic, leaving head intact. Do not remove all of the skin. Cut half an inch off the top of the garlic. Drizzle with olive oil. Sprinkle with salt and pepper. Bake on center rack for 40 minutes until garlic has softened. Remove from oven. Place on plate to cool. Once garlic has cooled, squeeze roasted garlic into a small bowl. The paste will be added to the soup.

In large saucepan or Dutch oven, heat 1/2 teaspoon olive oil. Add onion and celery and cook until softened, about 5 minutes. Stir in tomatoes and juice, 1 cup water and all seasonings. Bring to a boil. Reduce heat, add roasted garlic paste and simmer for 30 minutes. Purée with hand blender until mostly smooth. *(Note: You can save time and energy by roasting a few garlic bulbs at once. Roasted garlic is fabulous as part of many dishes, and even as a condiment or spread.)*

Nutritional information per serving:
71 calories; 2g protein; 3g fat; 11g carbohydrates.

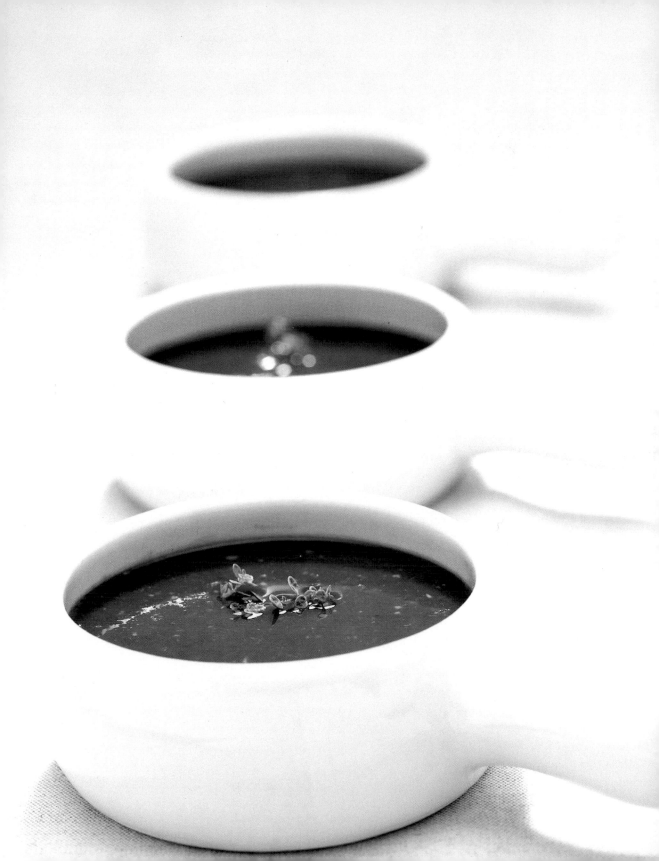

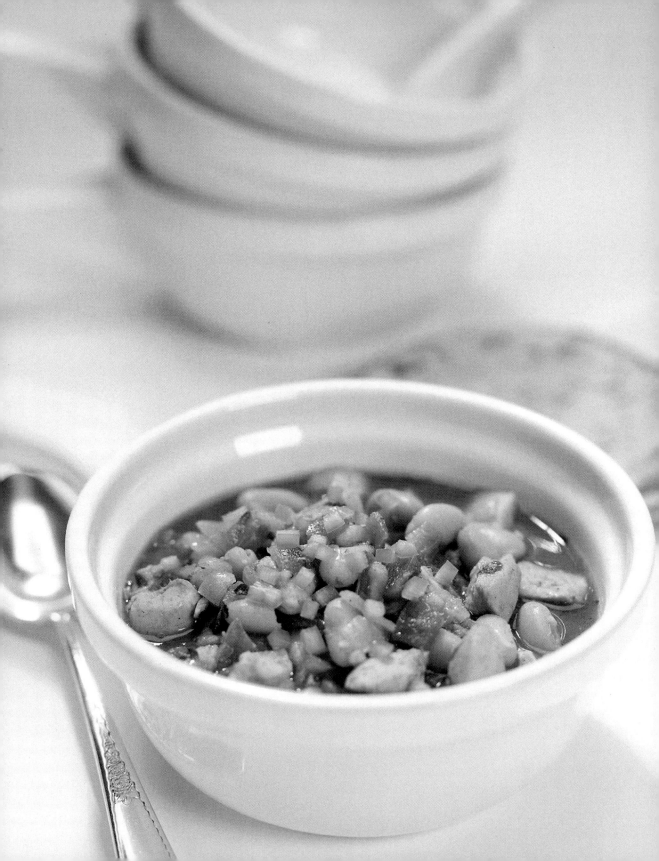

HEARTY WHITE
BEAN CHILI

. . . .

MAKES 6-8 SERVINGS

A thick chili served piping hot tastes wonderful no matter what the temperature outside. Using leaner cuts of poultry, including turkey or chicken breast, reduces the fat content but delivers a taste sensation.

INGREDIENTS

1 pound	dry great northern beans or white kidney beans, rinsed and picked over
4 cups	low-sodium chicken broth
2 cups	yellow onions, chopped
3 large	garlic cloves, minced
2 tsp	ground cumin
1½ tsp	dried oregano
1 tsp	dried ground coriander
⅛ tsp	ground cloves
1	(4-oz) can chopped green chilies
2 pounds	boneless, skinless chicken or turkey breast, grilled and cubed
1 tsp	sea salt

INSTRUCTIONS:

Place beans in a soup kettle or Dutch oven. Add enough water to cover beans by two inches. Bring to a boil. Let boil for 5 minutes. Remove from heat and let stand covered for 1 hour. Drain and rinse. Discard liquid.

Place beans in a slow cooker. Add the chicken broth, onions, garlic and seasonings. Cover and cook on low heat for seven hours or until beans are not quite tender. Add the chilies, chicken and sea salt. Cook for another hour until beans are tender.

Nutritional information per serving:
442 calories; 50g protein; 4g fat;
51g carbohydrates.

SWEET INCA PORRIDGE

. . . .

MAKES 4 SERVINGS

Quinoa, the humble grain revered by ancient Inca peoples, is enjoying a revival. Packed with more protein than any other, this crunchy yellow grain was referred to by the Inca as the "mother grain." Quinoa has more calcium than milk and is an excellent source of iron, phosphorus, B vitamins and vitamin E. Tip: Rinse quinoa with hot water, shaking vigorously to remove the bitter taste, before cooking.

INGREDIENTS

1 cup	quinoa grains, soaked
1 cup	rolled oats, not instant
¼ tsp	sea salt
3 cups	water
½ cup	chopped dates
1 tsp	nutmeg
1 tsp	cinnamon
1 tsp	best-quality vanilla

INSTRUCTIONS:

Place first four ingredients in pot with a tight-fitting lid. Cover. Bring to boil and then reduce heat to low. Simmer 30 minutes. Add remaining four ingredients and mix together well. Turn off heat and let sit, covered, for five minutes. Serve for breakfast with berries.

Nutritional information per serving:
315 calories; 9g protein; 4g fat;
62g carbohydrates.

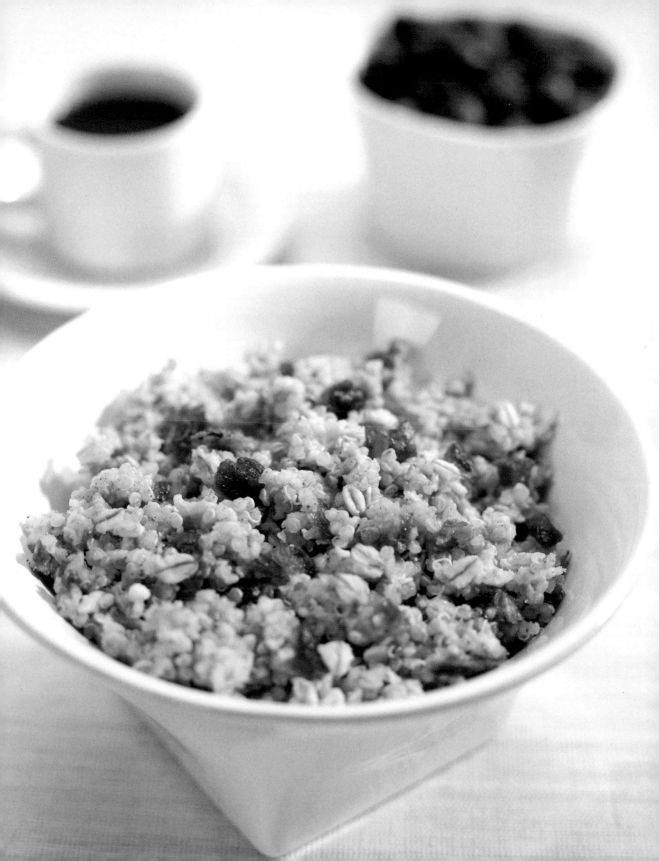

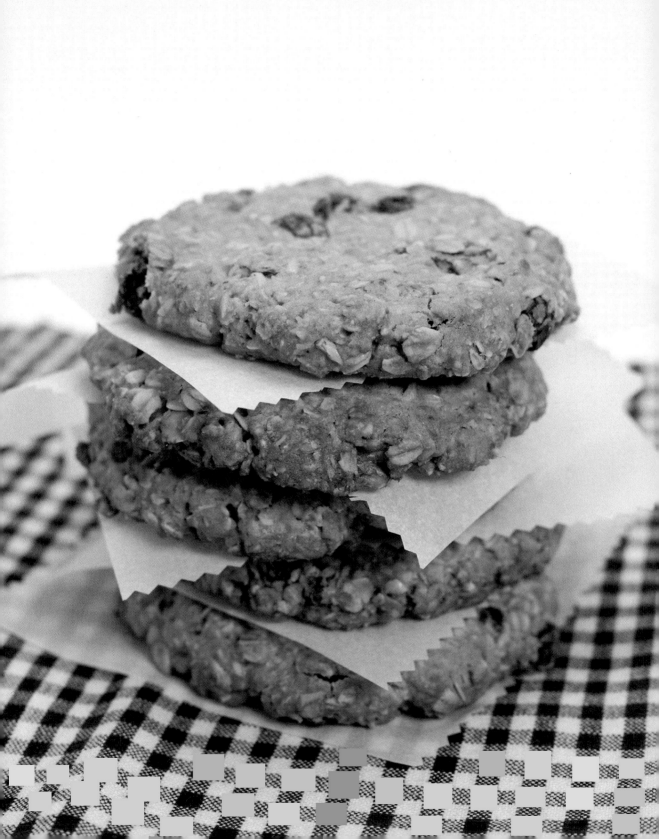

GRANDMOTHER'S FAVORITE
OATMEAL COOKIES

. . . .

MAKES 24 LARGE COOKIES

E very special occasion at our house is marked with the baking of these generous cookies. The batter is so hefty it requires a pair of clean hands to mix it. Best of all, they are not full of unnecessary sugar and they taste amazing. Everybody loves them! There are never any left over when the festivities are done.

INGREDIENTS

2⅔	cups unsalted olive-oil-based margarine
2 cups	packed brown sugar
3 large	omega-3 eggs
3 Tbsp	honey
1 Tbsp	best-quality vanilla
1½ tsp	sea salt
3 pounds *(8 cups)* old-fashioned rolled oats	
4 cups	unbleached all-purpose flour
8 oz	dark raisins *(optional)*
8 oz	coarsely chopped walnuts *(optional)*

INSTRUCTIONS:

Preheat oven to 350°F. Line baking sheets with parchment paper or Silpat sheets. Cream the margarine and sugar together in a large bowl until smooth. Beat in the eggs, honey, vanilla and sea salt until smooth and creamy. Use a large wooden spatula or your clean hands (best plan) to work in the flour and oats until well combined. Add raisins and walnuts if desired and mix until evenly distributed. Shape the dough into large three-inch balls and press into five- or six-inch flat cookies on baking sheets. Bake for 15 minutes or until as brown as you desire. Cool on wire racks. Make the cookies smaller if you like! Makes 24 very large and very delicious cookies.

*Nutritional information per cookie
(with raisins and walnuts):*
*471 calories; 6g protein; 27g fat;
52g carbohydrates.*

*Nutritional information per cookie
(without raisins and walnuts):*
*380 calories; 4g protein; 21g fat;
47g carbohydrates.*

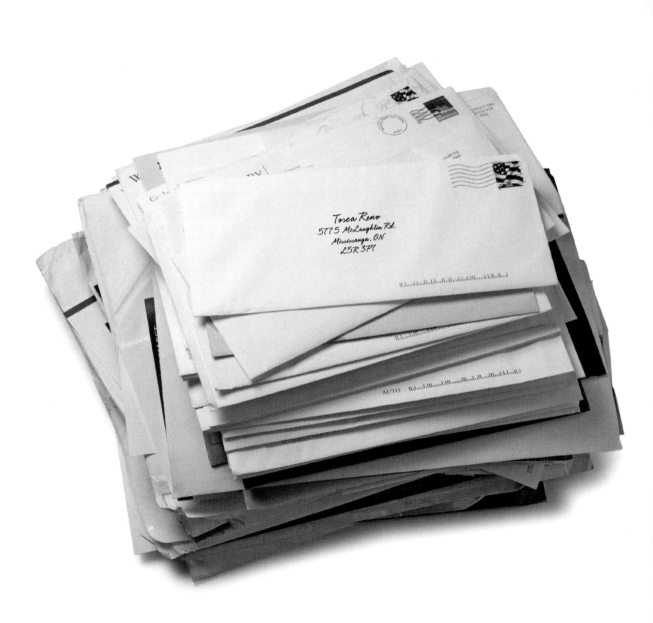

Tosca Reno
5775 McLaughlin Rd.
Mississauga, ON
L5R 3P1

CHAPTER FOURTEEN

CLEAN-EATING FAQ'S AND Q&A'S

WHAT'S THE BIG STINK ABOUT?

Q: I've just started to Eat Clean and, I'm embarrassed to say, I'm really gassy and bloated. Is this normal?

A: Yes, I'm afraid that reaction is quite common until you get used to the new way of eating. It's all the extra fiber and protein. However, you can help out by doing the following:

1. Chew chew chew! Whatever isn't broken down in your mouth must be broken down in your stomach. That creates lots of extra gas.

2. Drink tons of water.

3. Try products such as Beano. They do help, but you can't use them if you have a hard time with penicillin.

4. Take digestive enzymes or add some kefir to your diet. Both are inexpensive, natural, and very helpful because they add healthful bacteria to your digestive system.

And take heart. Once your body gets used to all this healthy food, your gas problem should calm down.

STRESSED OUT

Q: Can stress make me gain weight? I am overstressed at work, can't pay my bills on time and the kids and I are always fighting. I feel totally burnt out.

A: **Dr. Pamela Peeke, MD**, hit the bestseller list with a book called *Fight Fat After Forty*. She identified stress as a cause of obesity in many women. The hormone cortisol, which in the short term aids the body in mobilizing energy in stressful situations such as rushing a child to the ER, is cited as a cause of added fat on the body, particularly in the abdominal area. Too much cortisol apparently also decreases muscle mass and stimulates appetite. In fact, Cushing's syndrome, in which your body produces too much cortisol, is also known as the obesity disease. Whatever the case, constant stress is unhealthy. It upsets the thinking process and can cause ulcers and heart problems. You must take steps to reduce stress in your life. Try meditation or yoga. You will probably find there are courses in your area that teach you how to combat stress. And by the way, Clean Eating and regular exercise are very helpful in this regard.

ALCOHOL

Q: I need to lose weight and start Eating Clean, but I like my wine. Can I continue to drink alcohol?

A: It has been argued that some wines have advantageous properties. Certainly an occasional drink or two can relieve stress and induce relaxation, but since you want to lose weight I would not

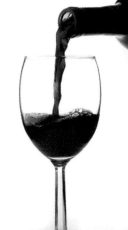

drink any alcohol at all. Not only is alcohol a sugar that packs on the pounds in no time, it reacts in your body in such a way that you have less energy to exercise properly, and it lowers your inhibitions. This means after drinking alcohol you are far more likely to indulge in decidedly non-clean foods.

Concentrate on Eating Clean and you will reach your goal. You will learn to do without alcohol, and feel much better for it.

JUICE FACTS

Q: **What is the truth about juice drinking? Is it good or bad?**

A: Remember when you had juice at breakfast only? Not any more. These days certain people (especially kids) grab juice out of the fridge all day long. They have juice boxes at school, on the playground and in the car. Juice drinking has become an around-the-clock habit that has gone too far. Apple juice has replaced milk, so many are now not getting sufficient calcium. Yes, juice comes from fruit, but it's not the same as eating a whole apple or orange. There's no fiber, only sugar calories with vitamins. Next time you're tempted to grab a glass of juice, go for the piece of fruit instead.

CALORIES DON'T COUNT

Q: **How many calories should I be eating each day? How many calories am I eating a day if I follow your menu plans?**

A: Calorie counting is not part of Eating Clean. It is an inaccurate science that does not account for the difference in how your body reacts to a calorie from a nutrient-rich food as it does to a nutrient-bereft food. Your body also reacts to calories differently depending on your metabolism, on how often you eat, etc.

What I dislike most about calorie counting is that it destroys our natural relationship with food. We get obsessed with numbers instead of what our bodies are telling us. Until about the middle of the last century, almost everyone was quite lean, and those who were overweight had nowhere near the obesity we see now. The obesity rates began to soar at just about the same time we all started counting calories. We know that dieting makes people fat, and in my opinion calorie counting does too.

Simply watch your portion sizes using your hands – lean protein is the size of your palm, complex carbs from whole grains or starchy vegetables is one cupped handful, complex carbs from veggies and fruit fits in two hands cupped together – and

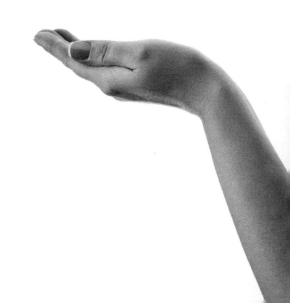

learn to listen to your body's natural signals of hunger and satiety. If you aren't hungry when your next mealtime comes, then decrease your portions slightly. If you are starving and you have an hour till your next meal, increase your portions slightly. Simple!

SLEEP DEPRIVED

Q: **How important is sleep in weight control? I have a night job and work odd hours. I find it hard to get the recommended eight hours' sleep each night.**

Regular sleep is important. Obesity has become an epidemic in this country and so has sleep deprivation. There could be a closer link than we first thought. In fact, the NSF (National Sleep Foundation) has stated: "Sleep deprivation is the royal route to obesity."

It doesn't take a genius to figure out that a person getting only four hours' sleep a night may not have enough energy to walk, let alone run or work out in a gym. But scientists have discovered even more ways sleep affects hunger. "If you limit the amount of time you are in a deep sleep, the brain interprets this as insufficiency of energy stores," says Jana Klauer, MD, a research fellow at the New York Obesity Research Center of St. Luke's-Roosevelt Hospital. "It thinks you are in a state of starvation" – and ups your appetite accordingly.

Lack of sleep can also cause your metabolism to slow down – another victory for obesity. In addition, when you are sleeping your body builds and repairs

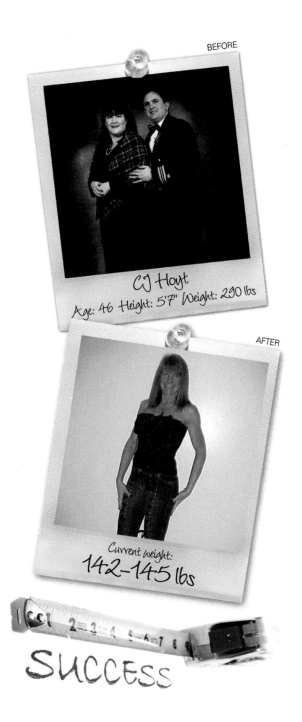

BEFORE

CJ Hoyt
Age: 46 Height: 5'7" Weight: 290 lbs

AFTER

Current weight:
142-145 lbs

SUCCESS

muscle tissue, which we already know burns the most calories. Your body also regulates hormones at night, and research has shown that the hormones that regulate fat burning and appetite – in particular carb cravings – get messed up when you don't sleep enough.

Of course even an eight-hour-a-night sleeper has to eat correctly and enjoy a certain amount of physical activity to keep weight levels under control. If it's impossible for you to get eight hours at one time, then take a nap or two through the day.

VEGETARIAN CLEAN EATING

Q: Can I follow this diet if I am a vegetarian/vegan?

A: You do not have to eat meat or eggs or any other animal product to Eat Clean. You just have to make sure you consume protein along with your complex carbohydrates at every meal. See page 25 for a list of high-protein foods from vegetable sources.

For meat-free Clean-Eating recipes, I use lots of tofu, which is great because it picks up the flavors of the other foods you cook it with. Cooking with tofu is like painting on a blank canvas. In addition I use many lentils, beans and quinoa – a highly nutritious, high-protein "grain" (really it's a seed, but it is used like a grain). I add edamame to soups, stews and pilafs. I also use textured vegetable protein, which is great as a replacement for ground meat in any recipe. I add hemp protein powder to my oatmeal and of course make protein shakes as well. I also

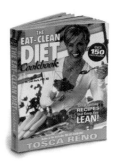

like Salba, or chia seed, another superfood with high protein.

I've also included many vegetarian recipes in *The Eat-Clean Diet Cookbook.*

FOOD ALLERGIES AND SENSITIVITIES

Q: Can I follow this diet if I have allergies or dietary restrictions?

A: Yes, the Eat-Clean lifestyle is very flexible and can be adapted to work with any dietary issues. Just follow the Eat-Clean principles and consume whichever foods you can.

So if you are allergic to gluten or can't eat seafood, no fear, just don't eat them!

BRAND OF PROTEIN

Q: Can you recommend a particular brand of protein powder or protein bars?

A: I choose not to recommend a specific brand because different areas have access to different products.

When picking a protein powder or bar, read the ingredients. Many protein bars are thinly disguised candy. You want to avoid chemicals, fillers and sweeteners. Also, check the amount of protein you get.

If you are lactose intolerant or vegan, there are many alternatives to whey protein you can use, such as soy or hemp protein.

For the most part, I don't really eat protein bars unless I am stuck without food for longer than anticipated. My favorite kind are the ones I make at home, and I've shared the recipe in *The Eat-Clean Diet Cookbook*.

CLEAN OR NOT CLEAN?

Q: **How do I know if a particular product is Clean?**

The most important way to see if a product is Clean is to read the ingredients. You always want to stay away from added chemicals and preservatives, added sugars and artificial sugars, too much salt, and unhealthy fats. If the words "hydrogenated" or "partially hydrogenated" occur, put the item back on the shelf. Clean food is anything nutritious that is as close as possible to how it occurs in nature.

Try not to get taken in by products that say "low fat" or "natural" on them. This doesn't always mean they are good for you. Read the ingredient and nutritional information carefully – serving sizes can often be misleading. I've read a label for fruit juice that only accounts for half of the single-serve bottle, and potato chip labels that give you the nutritional values for eight chips!

I think it's better to create your own meals as often as possible. That way you always know the ingredients and how fresh your food is.

NIGHT SHIFT

Q: **Can I live the Eat-Clean lifestyle if I work the night shift or shift work?**

A: The great thing about *The Eat-Clean Diet* is that it can be easily adapted to any lifestyle. Plan to eat five or six meals a day at two- to three-hour intervals. This goes for every day, whether you are working or not, and whatever time you wake up and go to bed.

For example, if you are having your first meal of the day at 3 pm, then your next meals would follow at approximately 6 pm, 9 pm, 12 am, and 3 am. Just try not to eat within about four hours of your bedtime, whenever that is, unless you are truly hungry.

Eat breakfast soon after you wake to start your day feeling energized and get your metabolism humming!

HATE TO COOK

Q: **Do I have to cook to Eat Clean?**

A: You don't have to cook to follow the Eat-Clean lifestyle, although I find it's easier to cook my own food so that I can ensure is 100% Clean rather than reading through labels all of the time.

Here are some easy tips to save on cooking:

❯ Keep raw, unsalted nuts and nut butter around. You can grab a piece of fruit and pair it with nuts for a complete Eat-Clean meal.

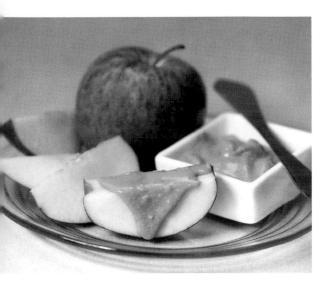

> Have whole-wheat, brown rice or Ezekiel wraps on hand. You can throw some cooked chicken breast, veggies and hummus in a wrap and you've got a great Clean meal.

> Cook large batches of food at one time. You can bake enough chicken breasts and boil enough eggs for a few days and keep them in the fridge. I also cook enough brown rice to last a few days. My daughter loves to make large batches of turkey meatballs to use on wraps, on Ezekiel bread hamburgers, or with salad and veggies.

> Keep raw veggies and fruits washed and ready in the fridge and on the counter. These can be tossed into a salad, used for wraps or eaten with some pre-made hummus or yogurt cheese. Buy prepackaged salads and keep them in your fridge.

> For breakfast you can have a hardboiled egg with some fruit, or eat Clean granola, muesli or oatmeal with some yogurt or cottage cheese and fresh or frozen berries for breakfast – a wonderful breakfast that requires no cooking.

You might have to cook a little, but if you plan and prepare in advance, cooking will be quick and easy.

EXACT MENU PLANS

Q: Do I have to follow the menu plans exactly? I don't like some of the items. Can I use different foods?

A: The meal plans I have provided in the book are merely suggestions. You can replace any of the foods, as long as you make sure to replace a complex carbohydrate with a complex carbohydrate and a lean protein with another lean protein. You don't have to eat something you don't like just because I've included it in the plan. Feel free to shake things up with some new recipes or by adapting old favorites to Clean recipes.

The Eat-Clean lifestyle is very flexible. Switch foods, or move different meals around to different parts of the day. Just remember to stick to the Eat-Clean principles and you'll be fine.

HOW LONG?

Q: How long will it take for me to see results?

A: When you begin the Eat-Clean lifestyle, you will find that you have more energy and that your skin and hair will become lustrous and healthy look-

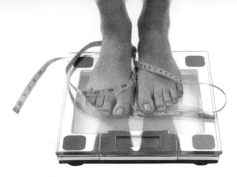

ing. This is the first sign that you are making a positive change to your health.

Each person will experience a different rate of weight loss. This is due to a number of factors such as starting weight, genetics, metabolism, the implementation of exercise, and how much you dedicate yourself to Eating Clean.

Healthy weight loss occurs at a rate of one to three pounds a week. Some weeks you'll lose more, some weeks you'll lose less and some weeks you might not see any movement at all. (But don't let that discourage you! Other positive changes are taking place in your body.)

This rate of loss allows your body to adjust to the changes. You might be surprised at the difference two pounds can make. Losing weight at this rate also helps your skin adjust, which helps to minimize the excess skin that you might have after you finish losing. Your heart, lungs and muscles also need a chance to catch up.

Also, let's not forget that the scale is inaccurate. The scale can't tell the difference between the fat lost and lean muscle mass gained. Your clothing size may get smaller and smaller while the numbers on the scale might stay put. I suggest using your body's measurements to keep track of your progress.

EAT-CLEAN PREGNANCY

Q: I'm pregnant. Can I follow the Eat-Clean lifestyle?

A: Eating Clean during your pregnancy is safe, but you should definitely check with your healthcare professional to ensure you are getting everything you need for you and your baby. You will need to pay attention to your calcium intake. Do not follow the cooler-one plan while pregnant.

NURSING MOM

Q: I am breastfeeding. Can I follow the Eat-Clean lifestyle?

A: Nursing moms burn more energy because they are producing milk. It's like a built-in baby-weight-loss machine!

You can certainly follow the Eat-Clean lifestyle and get in tune with your body. If you are honestly hungry after your sixth meal of the day, then go ahead and have a seventh. It's a flexible system as long as you are getting your nutrition every two to three hours and sticking to smaller portions. You don't want to starve your body of nutrients, especially at this time, so if you are hungry, EAT! And as with pregnancy, this is not a time for cooler one.

However, you should remain a vigilant Clean Eater with those late-night meals. Try to limit snacks to fresh sliced turkey or chicken breast, salt-free nuts, seeds, avocado, egg whites, berries, apples, carrots and celery.

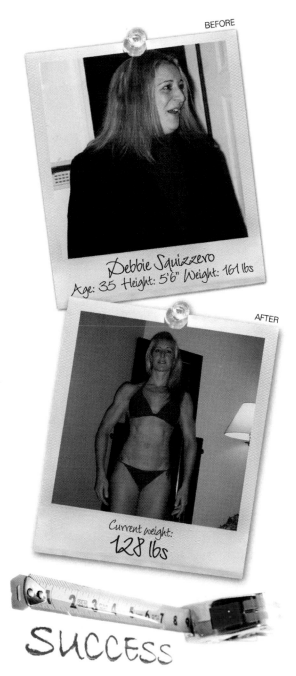

BEFORE

Debbie Squizzero
Age: 35 Height: 5'6" Weight: 161 lbs

AFTER

Current weight:
128 lbs

SUCCESS

Again, I encourage you to share this book with your health-care professional for his or her approval before following this plan.

LOTS OF WEIGHT TO LOSE

Q: I am severely overweight. Should I have gastric bypass surgery or liposuction? I'm not sure I can lose weight on my own.

A: Liposuction is not for the severely overweight. This surgical method of fat removal is really for those who are in good shape but have specific pockets of fat they have a hard time getting rid of — the lower belly region or upper thighs, for example.

Lap band and gastric bypass are both severe steps and should not be taken lightly. I hear from many people who have had gastric bypass who can never eat a normal-sized (not huge) meal ever again. Those with gastric bypass surgery will also have a hard time getting enough nutrients for the rest of their life. The lap band procedure is adjustable, and is better for getting nutrients once weight has been lost.

There are risks associated with both surgeries and with both of them the real key to success is not the surgery itself but rather the changes in eating habits, exercise, and the way you view food. I always feel that the natural way is best — in other words, using nutrition and exercise to lose all the excess weight. And you must keep in mind that even these operations are no magic bullet.

However, we are all individuals and some people need a little more help than others with certain problems. Be sure to talk to your physician about all your options and he/she will help you choose the one that's best for you.

DIABETIC

Q: Can I follow this diet if I have diabetes?

A: If you are thinking of following the Eat-Clean lifestyle, I urge you to discuss this program with your doctor. However, many health-care professionals have told me this is exactly how they think diabetics should eat, and I am certainly aware of many diabetics who use this program and whom it has helped.

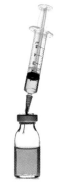

One of the reasons this program is so effective is that it regulates blood sugar. That's why I don't suffer from the effects of hypoglycemia anymore. However, I want to reiterate that I am not a doctor, so make sure to show the book to your doctor for approval.

TOO OLD?

Q: Am I too old to see a change if I start Eating Clean?

A: It is never too late to make a change for the better. Regardless of age, the Eat-Clean lifestyle can help you improve your health and physique. In fact,

I once received a wonderful letter from a woman in her 70s who had lost 75 pounds and become a fitness instructor.

TOO MUCH EATING!

Q: I don't think I can eat this much food. Is eating this way going to make me gain weight?

A: While it may seem like a lot of food, it's a lot of clean-burning fuel that your body needs. Your metabolism requires constant maintenance to stay steady throughout the day. It's like putting good-quality gas in your car to ensure it runs as best as it can.

That being said, if you find you are not hungry within three hours of your last meal, you can try slightly decreasing your portion sizes.

Whatever you do, don't skip meals. Just one skipped meal can tell your body to slow down its metabolism.

OTHER QUESTIONS

CHOCOHOLIC

Q: I have gotten into the habit of buying Kit Kat and Mars bars whenever I see them at a checkout counter. Time and time again I tell myself: "Just this one last time," but I realize that I've been doing this for years. I'm 44 years old and, yes, I'm obese but hate to admit it to anyone.

Jean R. Hackman
East Greenwich, RI

A: The trouble with habits is that the bad ones are harder to break than the good ones. You'll have to develop your willpower. This should help: try stripping off and truly looking at yourself in the mirror. Stop kidding yourself. You don't have to admit your obesity to anyone. It's there to be clearly seen by all.

Next time you are at the checkout counter grab a small packet of salt-free nuts instead of a candy bar. Or make sure you have your Eat-Clean cooler with you, so you always have a Clean option. Don't even look at the junk food when you approach the checkout station. You simply have to reinforce your desire to be slim.

COUNTRY GAL

Q: **I used to live in the city but now my husband and I have moved to the countryside. The grocery store where I live doesn't have a great variety of produce. How can I eat well if I'm so limited in my choices?**

Dotty Bell
Arthur, ON

A: Since you live in the country, you now have a huge supply of fresh vegetables and fruit. You should have plenty of roadside stands to get the freshest vegetables possible. Go to the local co-op and ask the owners which farmers sell produce, fresh eggs and poultry directly from their farm. You might encounter a world of freshness you never knew!

Also, the Internet is a great resource for foods that you cannot get at your local grocery store.

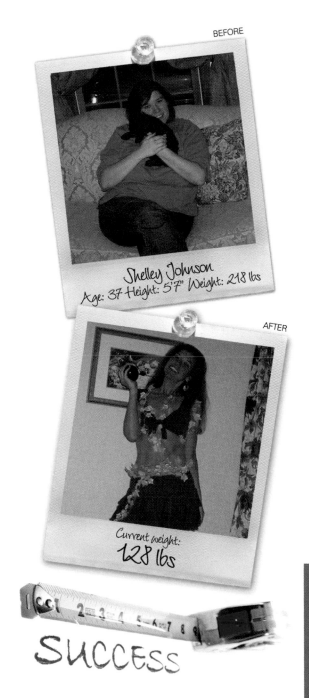

BEFORE

Shelley Johnson
Age: 37 Height: 5'7" Weight: 218 lbs

AFTER

Current weight:
128 lbs

SUCCESS

100 POUNDS OVER-WEIGHT

Q: **I am a fat slob. A trip to my bathroom scales this morning showed me that at 5' 5", I weigh 219 pounds. I am 100 pounds overweight. I've tried every diet around, lost a few pounds here and there but always gained back the weight and more. I feel like throwing in the towel and giving up. I will always be fat.**

Joyce Armstrong
Phoenix, NV

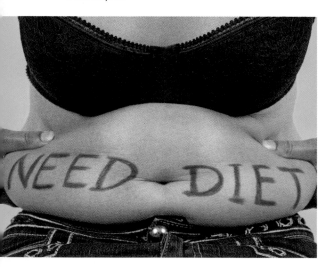

A: Your self-esteem is in the toilet. It will ultimately defeat you if you don't make steps in the right direction. You can try a zillion different diets and they'll never work. Clean Eating is a lifestyle change.

For the best results, you must do everything possible to maintain a positive attitude. This means you must be positive in how you think about yourself and how you reflect it in your speech and actions. Your final statement, "I will always be fat," is nothing but negative. Why not change that to "I will make a change and stick to it"?

Every day you must visualize how you want to look. Keep that image with you. Believe that it's possible – truly believe. And it is possible! Remember, I once weighed over 200 pounds, too. This positive attitude and belief in yourself combined with the mental image of how you want to look, will be all the incentive you need to modify your behavior and reach your weight-loss goals.

It has to be repeated: Clean Eating is a lifestyle change. You continue for the rest of your life. There is no doubt that your fat will come off. It won't happen in a day, a week or a month, but it will happen, and if you stay on course it will never come back. As for side effects, try these: you will be happier, healthier, fitter, and totally shocked at how awesome you look. Make it happen.

AGING PROCESS

Q: **I am 43 years old and I can see that age is catching up to me. Until recently, I have been a moderate smoker and drinker but now after reading *Oxygen* magazine (women's fitness), I have begun an exercise program. I feel better but I am still fearful of the aging process. Any answers?**

Ann McRobert
Albuquerque, NM

A: There was a disheartening article in *Esquire* magazine some time back. The article stated that we lose about one percent of our functional capacity every year after the age of 30. The author went on to suggest that our "best strategy may be simply to relax, and accept peacefully the indignities as they occur."

Yes, we are all aging but we don't have to decline by 10 percent each decade after the age of 30. Age isn't really aging, it's "rusting." If we exercise regularly, Eat Clean, avoid stress, and stay away from drugs, alcohol and tobacco, we are going to beat that one-percent-per-year statistic. I've seen it too many times to believe otherwise.

Age does slow us down. Wrinkles cannot be avoided. Loss of strength, endurance and flexibility is in the cards for all of us. But if we keep using our muscles, stretching our limbs; if we push our endurance and avoid drugs, tobacco and junk food, we challenge the statistics. We definitely push back the accepted aging process to a measurable degree.

HELP – I'M STARVING!

Q: **I'm so hungry by supper that I devour my food like a ravenous dog. I have been heavy since my teens and I can't seem to lose weight. I walk two miles a day and only have two meals a day, but I like my potato chips when I'm watching TV at night. I need help.**

Barb Shelby
Washington, DC

A: Forget the two big meals. You should be eating five or six smaller meals each day. Eat every meal slowly and never put more food on the plate or

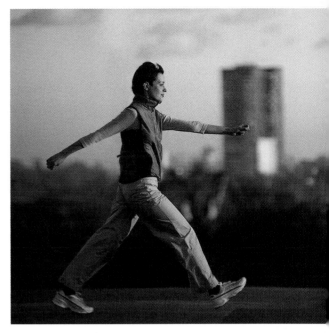

even on the table than you plan to eat. And sorry, but the potato chips have to go.

Include something at each meal that must be chewed for a long time. For example, a whole-grain cereal takes longer to eat than Corn Flakes or Special K. A large, raw carrot takes longer to eat than soggy canned vegetables. Your diet should consist of whole, natural foods that have all the bulk and fiber left in them, with no sugar added. Eat plenty of whole grains, fresh vegetables and fruit.

Once you start Eating Clean you will find that you are no longer ravenous at dinner. You will simply feel a healthy hunger.

Your habit of walking two miles a day is great. Walking is a good fat burner. Try adding some weight training and more strenuous cardio for better results.

DAIRY FOR WEIGHT LOSS?

Q: I have read that calcium from milk will help me lose weight. True or false?

Muriel V.
Hollywood, FL

A: If you are lacking calcium in the diet, then balancing the situation can do nothing but good. However, those who keep advocating consumption of milk to facilitate weight loss are usually folks with a financial interest in the area. All mammals start their lives with milk in order to gain weight, although admittedly we consume milk with most of the fat removed. It is a magic food, but evidence that it will do much good for those trying to lose body fat is extremely flimsy.

CALORIE BALANCE

Q: I read in a nutrition book that being overweight is simply a matter of balancing your caloric intake like a bank balance – calories-in and calories-out. Any excess gets stored around the hips and thighs like extra money stored in the bank account. (Although I always seem to have more in my fat bank than in my money bank!) The book said a pound of fat is made up of 3,500 calories and that if you take in this amount of calories you will gain one pound of fat, and it doesn't matter if the calories come from lean chicken and veggies or from ice cream and candy.

Robert J Villers
Houston, TX

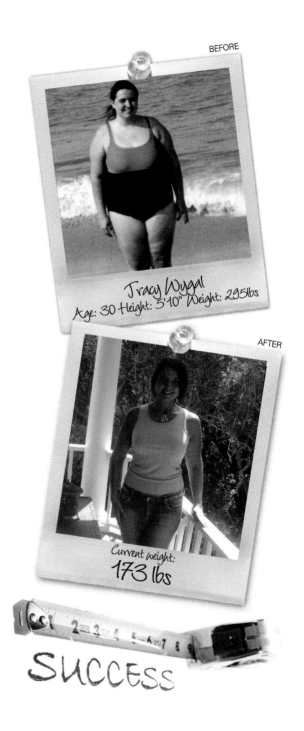

BEFORE

Tracy Wygal
Age: 30 Height: 5'10" Weight: 295lbs

AFTER

Current weight:
173 lbs

SUCCESS

A: I hope you threw out that nutrition book! Nothing could be further from the truth. The calories-in-calories-out theory is baloney. The body's appearance is made up from the food you eat. Consume junk such as candy, ice cream, potato chips, French fries and gravy, etc. and check out your body in the mirror a year from now. Conversely, Eat Clean for a year (veggies, fruits, lean meat, whole grains, fish and brown rice, etc.) and take a look. Not only will you look good, you will be considerably healthier. Years of junk-food consumption will lead to a depleted immune system and leave you open to a variety of serious illnesses. Eat Clean and you will be slim, energetic and healthy.

EXERCISE – THE TRUTH

Q: **I have heard that it is imperative to exercise if I want to lose weight. Please give me the truth.**
Remy Majors
Woodstock, NY

A: Here's your answer as you requested – the truth. You do not have to exercise if you want to lose weight. You can lose all the weight you desire by eating correctly. This is especially true for teenagers, who tend to have toned muscles underneath their fat. However, weight loss will occur more quickly if you exercise as well as follow a good diet. You hit the body from two angles and speedier results are inevitable.

There are of course greater advantages of exercise. Not only will you lose fat more quickly, but you will improve your energy, strength and fitness levels. You will also look better and improve your overall health if you exercise regularly. Consistent weight training will improve your physique by toning and shaping your body beyond your wildest dreams.

PROTEIN TO FAT

Q: **I know that protein is essential for building muscle, but can it also be converted into fat?**
JJ Woods
Thetford, Norfolk

A: Yup! An excess of any food that contains calories can be turned into fat. If you force yourself to eat an extra portion of lean chicken or steak every day, and you do not need those calories (energy), some of it will turn into fat.

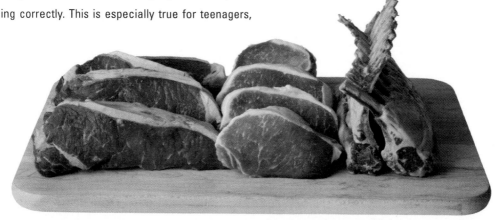

CREDITS

FRONT COVER PHOTO CREDIT
Paul Buceta (Make-up & hair by Lori Fabrizio)

BACK COVER PHOTO CREDIT
Robert Kennedy (Make-up & hair by Franca Tarullo)

INTERIOR PHOTO CREDITS
Paul Buceta (Make-up & hair by Franca Tarullo): page 14

Robert Kennedy: page 7, 31, 121 (*Tosca Reno* - **Make-up & hair by Franca Tarullo**)

Robert Reiff: pages 23 & 101, 34 & 70 (healthy plate), 54, 59, 79, 81, 83, 116, 198 (all excluding swordfish steaks), 199, 205, 206, 207, 210, 213, 216, 218, 221, 222, 225, 226, 232, 235, 236, 239, 240, 243, 244, 247, 248, (**Food styling credit- Janet Miller**)

Cory Sorensen: pages 26, 32, 33, 40, 64, 132, 134, 135, 145, 198 & 209 (swordfish steaks), 201, 202, 214, 217, 221, 229 (**Food styling credit- Ronnda Hamilton**)

Cathy Chatterton: pages 30 (*Tosca Reno* - **Make-up & hair by Franca Tarullo**), 60, 73, 109

Donna Griffith: page 108 & 230

All other photos from istockphoto.com